the family
in child health care

the family in child health care

Edited by

Pat Azarnoff, MEd
The Research Center
Wright Institute
Los Angeles

Carol Hardgrove, MA
Family Health Care Nursing
University of California
San Francisco

A WILEY MEDICAL PUBLICATION
JOHN WILEY & SONS
New York · Chichester · Brisbane · Toronto

Library of Congress Cataloging in Publication Data:

Association for the Care of Children's Health.
  The family in child health care.

  (A Wiley medical publication)
  Selected papers from the 14th annual international conference of the Association for the
Care of Children's Health.
  1. Sick children—Family relationships—Congresses. 2. Handicapped children—Family relationships—Congresses. 3. Parent and child—Congresses. 4. Child health services—Congresses.
I. Azarnoff, Pat. II. Hardgrove, Carol
III. Title. [DNLM: 1. Child, Hospitalized—Congresses. 2. Child health services—Congresses.
3. Family—Congresses. WS 105.5.H7 F198 1979]

RJ47.7.A87   1981   362.8'2   80-26586
ISBN 0-471-08663-0

Printed in the United States of America

10 9 8 7 6 5 4 3 2 1

contributors

Marvin Ack, PhD
Director of Human Ecology
Children's Health Center
Minneapolis, Minnesota

Association for the Care of Children's Health
3615 Wisconsin Avenue, N.W.
Washington, D.C.

Pat Azarnoff, MEd
Director, Pediatric Projects
Wright Institute Los Angeles
Los Angeles, California

Peg Belson
Founder and Executive Board Member
National Association for the Welfare of Children in Hospital
London, England

Bill S. Caldwell, PhD
Associate Professor, Department of Pediatrics
The University of Texas Medical Branch
Galveston, Texas

Dorothy Conway, RD, MPH
Assistant Professor, School of Public Health
University of Hawaii at Manoa
Honolulu, Hawaii

Catherine Daly, MSW, MPH
Instructor, School of Public Health
University of Hawaii at Manoa
Honolulu, Hawaii

Jessica G. Davis, MD
Director, Child Development Center Genetics Program
North Shore University Hospital
Manhasset, New York

Phyllis Eckert, MSW
High Risk Pregnancy and Perinatology Programs
North Shore University Hospital
Manhasset, New York

Donald H. Garrow, BM, FRCP
Consultant Pediatrician, Special Baby
    Care Unit
Wycombe General Hospital
High Wycombe, Bucks, England

Deborah Golden, MSW
Associate Project Director, Children and Youth Project
The University of Texas Medical Branch
Galveston, Texas

Bianca Gordon
Principal Psychotherapist
Greenwich & Bexley Area Health Authority
London, England

Carol Hardgrove, MA
Clinical Professor, Family Health Care Nursing
University of California School of Nursing
San Francisco, California

Maxene Johnston, RN, MA
Director, Ambulatory Services
Childrens Hospital of Los Angeles
Los Angeles, California

Calvin R. King, Jr., PhD
Assistant Professor, Department of Psychiatry and
    Behavioral Sciences
Medical University of South Carolina
Charleston, South Carolina

Barbara Korsch, MD
Professor of Pediatrics, School of Medicine
University of Southern California
Los Angeles, California

Ira Kurland, MSW
Clinical Social Worker
Childrens Hospital of Los Angeles
Los Angeles, California

Michael A. Lazarus, BA
Wantagh, New York

John Lind, MD
Professor Emeritus
Karolinska Institute
Stockholm, Sweden

Ivonny Lindquist
Head of Section
National Board of Health and Welfare
Stockholm, Sweden

Susan L. McMillan, PhD
Assistant Professor, Department of Pediatrics
The University of Texas Medical Branch
Galveston, Texas

Katherine O'Reilly, MPH
Assistant Project Specialist, School of Public Health
University of Hawaii at Manoa
Honolulu, Hawaii

Janet Payne, ACSW
Department of Mental Health and Mental Retardation
Memphis Mental Health Institute
Memphis, Tennessee

Audrey M. Rath, RN, MS
Nurse Practitioner Consultant
Arizona State Board of Nursing
Phoenix, Arizona

Marilyn Savedra, DNS
Assistant Professor, School of Nursing
University of California, San Francisco
San Francisco, California

Ann R. Sloat, RN, MSN
Assistant Professor, School of Public Health
University of Hawaii at Manoa
Honolulu, Hawaii

Roy Smith, MD, MPH
Professor, School of Public Health
University of Hawaii at Manoa
Honolulu, Hawaii

Lorraine Stringfellow, RN, BSN, MPH
Assistant Professor, School of Public Health
University of Hawaii at Manoa
Honolulu, Hawaii

Blanche B. Valancy, ACSW
Social Worker, Division of Child Neurology
Cleveland Metropolitan General Hospital
Cleveland, Ohio

Linda Williams, BA
Parent Consultant
American Heart Association
Long Beach, California

Richard Wittner, MD
Director of Pediatric Cardiology
Earl and Loraine Miller Children's Hospital Medical Center
Long Beach, California

preface

When a child is hospitalized, the impact on the family is immediate and long-lasting. Relationships and support systems change, power and authority shift from family to hospital personnel, and familiar guidelines disappear. This book examines in detail the effects these changes have on family life when the ill or disabled child is cared for in the hospital or outpatient health care setting.

The Family in Child Health Care brings special concerns about families to the attention of a variety of professionals, both pre-service and in-service. In the areas of health sciences and mental health it will be of interest to nurses and physicians, especially those in pediatrics; to play specialists in hospital and clinic playroom programs; to parent counselors and family advocates, members of a rapidly developing profession; to pediatric psychologists and child psychiatrists; and to teachers in preschool and primary classes who want to assist their students in coping with stressful medical encounters. Students of social systems and family dynamics will find the detail and provocative questions that will help them to develop a philosophy of care. The book will also be useful to parents, whether or not they belong to one of the many parent organizations of informed and active consumers, and to those agencies that advise them about their rights and about how to cope with a system that is supposed to help their children. In the international community, we welcome the interest of our colleagues in Canada, England, Sweden, and Australia particularly, since this work indicates that an interest in family programs has developed in these countries as well as in the United States.

Some recognized practitioners in this field are published in this collection for the first time. Others, who are acknowledged leaders in family care, present new work here. Issues of great interest and concern in the clinical area, which have not been published widely elsewhere, are discussed; for example, differences between parent-led and professionally-led parent groups, the stereotypes of "culture" unique to pediatrics, the dynamics of parent-inclusive units, and the effects on family interaction of "survivors," children who live through diseases that used to be terminal.

The papers that constitute the chapters in this collection were drawn from the fourteenth annual international conference of an educational and advocacy organization for humanizing health care for children and their families, now called the Association for the Care of Children's Health. ACCH has long encouraged the presentation of models of care through its journal, newsletter, and other publications as well as in affiliate educational sessions and annual international conferences. Through many advocacy efforts, the association has helped change pediatric policy and heightened awareness about family health care. ACCH performs these services in the belief that thoughtful intervention by members of the health care team during this sensitive period in the life of the family can encourage its growth and enhance its development.

It is our hope that this book will inspire readers to encourage family participation so that the child, the family, and the health care system will all benefit.

P. A.
C. H.

acknowledgments

Many people were helpful and supportive throughout the development of this work. Carlene Reuscher and David Rigler capably chaired the committees that selected topics and speakers for the conference from which these papers were selected. Patricia Anderson, Beverley Johnson, Gene Stanford, and Linda Williams, of the Association for the Care of Children's Health (ACCH), have encouraged our efforts to highlight the issues that families encounter in child health care. Hedda Bolgar, Director of Wright Institute Los Angeles, has long believed in the importance of studying and helping victims of social systems and was inspirational to us. Anita King, of the National Institute of Mental Health, has effectively supported our advocacy and research efforts with children and families.

We especially thank the contributors who have shared their work, ideas, experience, and insights in this volume.

We are grateful for the many hours and quality work of our staff: Virginia Lewis, grammarian and word processor par excellence, sensitively coordinated the contributor/editor communication; Mary Ann Indreland efficiently transcribed the tape recordings.

The agencies that cohosted the conference for ACCH are Wright Institute Los Angeles, a social action, education, and research facility whose focus is social-clinical psychology; Childrens Hospital of Los Angeles; Earl and Loraine Miller Children's Hospital Medical Center, Long Beach, California; and the Southern California Affiliate of ACCH.

This publication was supported in part by grants to the Wright Institute Los Angeles, LMO3214 from the National Library of Medicine and MH31404 from the National Institute of Mental Health.

Special thanks to Roy, Julie, LaMar, Karen, and Moshe and to Jim, Barbara, Sally, Steve, and Ann for family love and caring.

P. A.
C. H.

contents

the family
in child health care

INTRODUCTION

the family
in pediatrics

CAROL HARDGROVE AND PAT AZARNOFF

Carol Hardgrove, MA, Clinical Professor, Department of Family Health Care Nursing, the University of California, San Francisco, has served on the Executive Board of ACCH.

Pat Azarnoff, MEd, Director, Pediatric Projects, The Research Center, Wright Institute Los Angeles, coordinated the fourteenth annual ACCH conference and is a former president of the association.

This collection describes child health care from an era in which parents and siblings were excluded from the sick child's hospital room to an era in which parents have total care of the child and some control of the environment. This book represents the new thinking emerging in health care. The focus on the family, rather than solely on the child patient, generates from the belief that the child's illness is the family's illness, that the child's disability affects interactions in the entire family.

3

When health staff fully appreciate the impact of the child's illness or disability on the family and the effect of the family on the child, they provide programs to foster family closeness and encourage parents to give and accept emotional support.

IN THE PAST

The involvement of the family in the health care of the ill child has not always been welcome. Families have been barred from close contact with their child by hospital edicts. As late as 1964 many hospitals in the United States permitted visiting only twice a week for an hour at a time. When children cried at their parents' departure, both professionals and parents were convinced that the bedlam resulting from such visits was harder on the children than no visits at all. Many people perceived the desire of parents and children to be together as being somewhat neurotic, either evidence of overprotectiveness and spoiling or indication of parental lack of trust and respect for the medical and nursing staff.

Ordinarily, stories of a child torn from the arms of a mother move us to sorrow or indignation. Yet for many years hospitals were the agents of such outrages by routinely separating parents from their children. Weak attachments between parent and child were strained to the breaking point by such policies of estrangement perpetrated in the name of health care. The natural affection of parents and their concern for the continuation of routines familiar to the child was considered unreasonable and foolish coddling. Some staff members even took responsibility for breaking children's "bad habits," such as thumb-sucking, clinging to an old blanket, crying "unnecessarily," and indulging in messy eating and food preferences. In the interest of good care, nurses were supposed to be able to feed babies much better than mothers could. Breast-feeding of a sick baby was discouraged; instead the baby was weaned from the mother abruptly. Many professionals believed that the newborn and young infant were undiscriminating about caregivers and would therefore thrive even with minimal and random stimulation. Although it was eventually accepted that holding and cuddling are important, it was thought that anyone could provide this stimulation. It was thought that children quickly forgot their distress and were unaffected by the separation. Denying the importance of the family-child bonds, most staff appeared to believe that a hospital separation was not harmful.

Parents took great care not to offend the staff by questioning these policies, by appearing to be too close to their child, or by knowing too much. They feared that if they displeased the staff in whose hands their child's well-being rested, revenge on the child might result or care might be withheld.

People who grew up in that era have stories to tell about the heartbreak and even lifelong physical or emotional problems that stemmed from such treatment. After all, separating children from their familiar routines, from known surroundings, and from loved ones is seen as punishment. Although not intended by the staff, separation was interpreted by children as punishment.

IN THE PRESENT

Even though research has for some time shown that children were left with psychological scars and that families were disrupted, progress toward policies of emotional care has been random and uneven. New programs have begun to emerge that provide more attention to play, more frequent visiting, and preparation for potentially stressful events. Progress is slow in these areas, unlike the action that characteristically follows medical scientific discoveries.

It was found that babies and preschoolers who are developmentally vulnerable are psychologically at risk. With inadequate defenses and memory they are unable to cope with the strange, painful new surroundings without consistent, familiar nurturing. They cannot express either playfulness or pain without the presence of a trusted adult companion. Since young children are unable to put into words the trauma they experience, their reactions of fear and anger flare up after their return home. When play opportunities are provided in the health center, however, children explore unfamiliar items used on them by others and express feelings, release tension, and understand more about what is happening.

School-age children were found so likely to be disturbed by hospitalization that behavior disorders typically followed discharge from hospitals without psychosocial care. In addition, there were reports of delayed language development, learning difficulties, and lowered self-esteem. There are now a number of hospitals that welcome school groups on tours, offer preadmission orientation to patients and parents, and provide books, puppets, or other materials that add to the child's understanding and reduce the threat of the hospital environment.

Adolescents in health care were seriously affected by the feeling of vulnerability, the unfilled need to talk with someone about their future, and their fears about reactions from peers. With more adolescent units available and a greater understanding of the different nature of care needed for adolescents, more health centers are providing staff and programs especially designed for them.

Territorial imperatives of the staff were found to convey to parents that children belonged to the home culture only until they were hospitalized. Once admitted, the child magically belonged to the hospital culture. Those parents who tried to be supportive at the hospital found that when they were deprived of this role they could not easily resume their home relationships after the child was discharged; concepts of themselves as useful and appropriate caregivers were damaged. When parents are encouraged to continue the parenting role in the hospital they are able to provide the continuity and physical closeness that help children feel cared for. Parents bring their child's favorite items from home, offer closeness, and promote children's feelings of belonging, of being all-important to the family. A deeper attachment grows between parents and children.

Some hospitals that still discourage parents throw open their doors to clowns, baseball heroes, youth groups for parties, movie stars and television personalities seeking media exposure, community groups with used holiday cards, and volunteers with donated toys. These multiple strange contacts do not prevent the psychological damage in children they are intended to counteract. Indeed, these strangers may add stress to the child who is already overwhelmed by technology, machinery, and change. When parents are more welcome in hospitals, however, children can manage better. The presence of parents in a protective and guiding role can be reassuring to children and help them believe in their ability to learn and grow sturdier from their encounters with people and procedures in the health care system.

When the parent is accessible the child is found to tolerate sickness, pain, and frightening medical or surgical procedures with less immediate and long-lasting upset. It is not only the parents' explanations but also their actual presence that cushions and detoxifies the stressful experience and promotes recovery. Parents can also provide staff with a social and psychological history as well as a medical history, since they have intimate knowledge of the child's coping strengths in previous hospitalizations or clinic visits. The parents know if the child has had other recent losses such as the death of a relative or a pet, a recent move to a new home, or the birth of a sibling.

Parents as well as children need emotional care. In mutual-support groups parents help each other through the difficult times and with the management of the daily, practical aspects of long-term disabilities and chronic care. When the staff prepares families for the encounter in the health center, parents and patient are better able to comply with medical advice and there is greater trust and more satisfaction with the care.

Gaining the family's trust usually results in gaining the child's trust and decreases physiologic and psychologic distress. The family's trust also helps the staff to feel more satisfaction and enables them to avoid dissociating themselves from their own compassion. Examining an infant on the mother's lap instead of on an examination table, for instance, is easier not only on the baby, who is less fearful and defensive, but also on the staff who do not need to hold down or swaddle a terrified, struggling child, and who can enjoy a more appealing and curious one.

Attempting to treat the child without considering the family is now more often considered an exercise in futility. Health centers increasingly see the family's participation as crucial to the patient's recovery, especially when the longer-term effects on children's behavior are considered. Any hospital that sets policy to deprive parents and children of each other's company and comfort denies the vast literature on the benefits of family support and the deficits of separation.

As we look to health care in the future it is clear that most illnesses and disabilities will be treated in outpatient and home settings, combining the benefits of modern medicine with the virtues of home care. There will still be a need for emotional support and teaching but in varying formats. For example, the captive family waiting in a clinic may use the time to learn from materials developed in their language that speak to contemporary family concerns and acknowledge cultural values. Regular play demonstrations and observations may help them know more about their children and about family interactions. In the clinic or hospital parents will remain in need of nurturing, especially the increasing number who are themselves still adolescents with babies. Those who are struggling to rear families as single parents, those who are from a cultural or ethnic group different from that of the staff, and those who are unable to stay with their children will also need emotional support.

THE NEW THINKING

As health centers attempt to make needed changes to be responsive to children's distress and to include parents in care more often and more effectively they find the task is greater than opening the door and saying, "Come be with your child." The old ideas have become so ingrained that today many hospitals that have changed policies in light of the newer research face the challenge of wooing families into staying and helping with their children.

It is interesting to note from the papers in this book the expanded effort health and mental health professionals are making to reach out to families. These people are attempting to be attentive listeners and enablers, to learn from parents, and to see families engaged in mutual-help groups and becoming more assertive consumers. Here is a sampling of some of the practices that are emerging from the new thinking.

New Supports for Parents of Children in Health Care

• Preparation materials and activities.
• Education for parenthood of chronically ill children.
• Earlier psychosocial intervention.
• Intakes that include psychosocial status and cultural beliefs.
• Housing in or near the hospital at nominal cost or free.
• Vouchers for travel and food.
• Facilities for parents to cook familiar foods.
• Temporary but consistent parent substitutes, such as Foster Grandparents, for children whose parents cannot visit.
• Child care for well siblings during parent visiting of inpatients or during outpatient appointments.
• Sibling support groups.
• Advocacy from governmental agencies and hospital administrations.

New Roles for Families

• Nursing care in the hospital.
• Psychological support for the ill child.
• Home treatment, such as dialysis, chemotherapy, transfusions, injections.
• Staying with the child during anesthesia induction, in the recovery room, and in the intensive care unit.

New Roles for Health and Mental Health Professionals

• Coordinator of parent programs and groups.
• Specialist in family preparation for hospitalization.

- Coordinator of play programs in the hospital, clinic, and community health center.
- Family advocate.
- Postdischarge care coordinator.
- Home visitor.
- Family aide.

New Locations for Emotional Care of Families

- Hospice.
- Emergency room.
- Intensive care unit.
- Delivery room and other birth centers, home birth.
- Recovery room.
- At home or hospital for preadmission visits.
- Presurgical play/waiting room.
- Halfway house for children in day treatment.
- Family participation unit.
- Dormitory or house for parents of long-term or seriously ill children.
- One-day surgical unit.

RECOMMENDATION

We recommend a regular staff position of coordinator of family programs, an advocate who can seek out vulnerable families for care and encourage colleagues, despite staff turnover or cost factors, to continue to believe in family inclusion policies.

Coordinators can arrange for food service personnel to open small kitchens where parents may cook familiar dishes or special treats for their children. They can advise architects on the design of space and beds for parents of babies, young children, and critically ill older children to stay overnight or to rest during the day;

no one would be expected to get a night's rest in a chair. Coordinators can collaborate with nurses in teaching parents to give treatments they will have to continue at home. They can press for social workers to have smaller caseloads so that they can attend more fully to the emotional crises and not be given only financial and transportation concerns at the last minute. And they can generate play programs in every part of the health center that serves children.

Coordinators can bring help to the ordinarily well-functioning family who needs support during the immediate crisis and to the family whose prior dysfunction is seriously strained even by a minor, treatable illness. The coordinators can encourage families to support and teach each other.

In these and other ways, coordinators of family programs can look at the entire encounter in the health center, from preadmission to x-ray to discharge and follow-up. Coordinators can seek to collaboratively design a continuous support system for families and staff.

With this changing philosophy of family support, we must now apply the same amount of energy and commitment to welcoming and encouraging families as we formerly spent substituting for them.

It is the shared belief of the authors presented in this collection that the patient comes to health care as part of a family. These writers believe that there are a variety of methods for achieving the goal of strengthening the family through the fullest and most compassionate use of our institutions and ourselves.

We are hopeful that the creative and useful studies and models presented here will inspire, inform, and assist readers in their own efforts toward family-centered caring.

part I
ISSUES OF THE FAMILY
IN HEALTH CARE

PARENTS AND CHILDREN: CONFLICT AND CARING

1

the familiar stranger

BIANCA GORDON

Bianca Gordon serves as the principal psychotherapist for the Greenwich and Bexley Area Health Authority and offers consultation to many professionals and students regarding mental health issues that affect children and families. She has been involved in the child guidance movement in the United Kingdom. She encourages the practice of total care, which does not treat mind and body as separate entities, and suggests ways that parents and children can have emotional support in the hospital.

I have been involved in the care of sick children for many years and have become particularly aware of the emotional stress that they and their parents undergo. Consequently, I am concerned that academic knowledge about the needs of both children and parents find practical application in our hospitals. Seven-year-old Simon has simply and yet powerfully pinpointed the problems addressed in this paper. "They looked into my mouth and into my ears; they looked into my eyes, and they touched my tummy, but they never looked at me."

This is not to suggest, of course, that no attempt has yet been made to deal with the emotional needs of sick children. But we still have a very long way to go before a satisfactory situation is achieved.

The treatment of sick children should take into account their physical and emotional environment, including relationships with their families. Such total care cannot depend upon the efforts of any one department but requires interdisciplinary work. We need to concern ourselves with the emotional needs of the individual child who is still, far too often, a familiar stranger in our hospital units.

It is now more widely recognized that the hospital environment has an inevitable impact for better or worse, not only on children's immediate prospects of recovery, but also on their long-term emotional development. That children should not be separated from their families during hospitalization is now generally accepted in theory. But one particular aspect of the study of separation problems has yet to be further studied—that separation can be particularly harmful during the early weeks and months of the baby's life when there is still a biological bond between the baby and the mother.

Until recently, fulfillment of bodily needs was thought to be the dominant or even sole requirement in the first six months of life. Classical psychoanalysts believed that a suitable mother-substitute could satisfy these needs. But there is now much evidence that the baby experiences emotional dependence on his mother from the very beginnng and is, therefore, much affected by separation from her. We also know that the mother can suffer acutely from the baby's absence. This can lead to an estrangement that may have far-reaching consequences for their future relationship and for the baby's emotional development. Yet separation is part of life; a child has to cope with it at weaning, when walking begins, and later when school begins. Although separation is a natural process that starts from the moment of birth, the manner in which children have been helped to cope with it will have a bearing on their ability to deal with the hospital experience. Whether the hospitalization will harm a particular child may therefore depend on the quality of that child's relationship with the mother, as well as on the kind of previous experiences of being parted from her. It will not solely depend on the impact of the stay in hospital.

INDIVIDUALIZED ASPECTS OF SEPARATION

There are, of course, circumstances in which separation and illness can actually benefit children, especially when their relationships at home have contributed to the medical condition. Children from an insecure, troubled home may actually use the illness and the hospital experience to establish identity. Children who lack confidence in their relationship with their mothers may show this by making endless demands during visits.

Problems within the family circle tend to find echoes in the ward. A child's distress about matrimonial disharmony, for example, can be pathetically clear. One boy desperately ill with ulcerative colitis found his estranged parents reunited around his bed. Thus the illness, directly linked to his extreme anxiety over his parents, showed itself in his desperate wish to keep them by his bedside. He used his illness to reestablish his family as it once was. What matters more than the fact of separation, therefore, is its meaning to the individual child, and this would depend on the child's personality and the relationships within the family.

Separating children from normal environments produces significant and sometimes traumatic effects. We must not be satisfied with understanding the emotional problems of children in hospital in terms of separation only. Many of the children's emotional difficulties may relate less to this separation than to their illnesses. We must always bear in mind that the children are ill, and it is this fact, no less than separation, that changes their emotional needs, particularly those relating to their dependency. Children may regress, become hostile, depressed, listless, and withdrawn during an acute illness, whether looked after in a hospital or at home.

EMOTIONAL SUPPORT FROM PARENTS

The inevitable regression associated with illness has a significant effect on the child. Clinical work based on dynamic psychological theories provides fundamental insights that have application not only to certain individual patients, but to all children undergoing medical or surgical treatment. The all-important task of giving a child effective and consistent emotional support can only be achieved through a sustained personal relationship. Effective emotional support requires not only a sympathetic attitude but also knowledge of what it means to children to be forced by this illness to surrender some or all of their proudly acquired functions. The mastery of bodily functions such as eating, urination, defecation, and learning to wash are important milestones in children's lives. The surrender of these functions to others may be experienced as a powerful backward step. Some children, however, adjust without any apparent difficulty; others submit in a totally passive manner. Still others fight against helplessness and are ashamed of their physical weakness and of returning to dependency on adult help that they had just outgrown.

Understanding and gentle handling is needed to help these children retain their earlier self-image of the active and controlled child. Staff personnel need to anticipate that curtailment of motor activity may cause children to become frustrated, angry, and aggressive. Healthy children have ample opportunity for the necessary discharge of energy; when deprived of motility children must be provided with other outlets for their energy through words and play. Above all, young children need constant emotional support, since they are separated from familiar surroundings and suffer both the mental and physical stress of illness.

DANGERS OF EXCESSIVE FREEDOM

Care must be taken that the sense of being emotionally supported is not lessened by the relatively free and easygoing atmosphere that prevails in some of our modern progressive pediatric wards. The freedom given there must not create confusion in the minds of children about the identity of the supporting person.

In addition to sustained emotional support, very sick children need privacy and quiet. It is often difficult to provide these in some modern pediatric establishments that have changed from institutions with a rigid pattern of procedure to an environment almost too free to give the emotional support and security needed. Thus children's confusion may be increased in wards where staff no longer wear uniforms and where the identity of position cannot easily be recognized.

Just as regimentation and lack of reasonable freedom will have a stifling effect on sick children, so will too great a measure of freedom. This freedom carries with it the danger of making them unsure of their position in hospital and uncertain about what to expect and on whom to rely. There is much evidence that suggests that young children may interpret the well-intentioned freedom they are given in a hospital as a noncaring lack of interest on the part of those looking after them. The fun-and-games atmosphere of some of these wards can be a threat to children in severe pain, especially when they are very sick, dying, or under the impact of acute fears. Children may easily feel bewildered and isolated in an active but unstructured environment that is out of tune with their inner feelings. Children may even wish that staff would restrain them from giving free expression to instinctual but socially unacceptable behavior. Excessive freedom can deprive children of the points of reference, both place and time, that are especially necessary now that they are sick and torn away from familiar settings. Even more than healthy children, ill children look for signposts because they need to know where things are and when things happen. If there are no points of reference, children will experience inner chaos. It is, therefore, important for sick children to enter a sound and stable atmosphere. The difficulty in achieving this in a ward where the staff are frequently changing lays a special responsibility on such key figures as the senior physician, the head nurse, the teacher, and the play specialist. It falls on them to create and maintain a stable environment.

CHILDREN'S VIEW OF HOSPITAL

When taken to the hospital children may feel abandoned. Clearly defined routines of waking, eating, visiting, and sleeping will help to fill the void and help them cope with fears of having been deserted. Even so, fantasy and reality may still remain confused and the concept of time may be elusive.

The length of an illness or stay in hospital has a significantly different meaning for children than for the adults who take care of them. Children are likely to perceive a stay in hospital as a kind of imprisonment. Having to diet, being confined to bed, or being physically restricted can seem like an unending state of captivity, regardless of whether the stay is one day, two weeks, or longer. Children's perceptions of the passing of time is relative to the urgency and strength of their wishes and impulses. Even a short stay in the hospital can cause an almost unendurable frustration. Children may find postponing the fulfillment of a wish most difficult to bear. This applies to the gratification of an intellectual wish, such as the desire for the relief from pain and fear, or for affection, comfort, company, activity, or entertainment. It is vital for those taking care of sick children to understand these frustrations so that they will not dismiss children's reactions as unreasonable, behave unsympathetically, or fail to appreciate the degree of children's fretting. In light of this, it will readily be understood that remarks such as "Your mother will be here soon," or "Soon you will go home," do not really reassure. These assurances may, in fact, lead to mistrust if they turn out to be empty promises. Because the unfamiliar hospital environment is bound to appear strange and frightening, it is even more important to help children feel safe and secure. Children especially need to be reassured when they are in a state of physical discomfort and need help dealing with their fears and experiences that even sick adults would find hard to manage. Particular care should be taken to help children cope with feelings of imprisonment; it should be made easier for children to go home as soon as they are well enough without having to wait for what seems an interminable time.

It can be a severe shock to a child to find that his body suddenly is not the mother's concern but rather the concern of complete strangers. He cannot understand why, at a time when his emotional need for her is greatest, his body is looked at, handled, and sometimes hurt by those with whom he has not yet established a personal relationship. Children dislike having their bodies exposed and all the more so when on traction or in a burns unit.

Children ask to be covered because the desire for coziness and for privacy is very strong at such times. They have these desires especially when they are worried about what is happening and are bewildered by the many different people who attend day and night, and with whom they are expected to relate. It is hard for a child to accept that he is only one of many patients when what he needs most is to be treated as someone very special.

Physical pain is part of life, and children need loving support and praise in order to bear it. Unsupported, pain can be a traumatic experience for the child that can disturb future personality development. Excessive pain may well be especially harmful to an infant during the first year of life, even more than later on. Well-being depends on an optimum balance between pleasurable and painful experiences. When there is too much pain, when the unpleasurable experiences outweigh the pleasurable ones, this balance is disturbed, and reactions to the world around can change from hitherto trusting and open attitudes to suspicious and withdrawn ones.

ENCOURAGEMENT OF EXPRESSION

Ideally, a child should perceive the hospital as an extension of home, the only difference being that the hospital is better equipped to make him well quickly. To give children this sense of comfort and security, a sympathetic worker who does not inhibit but rather encourages the expression of worrying thoughts is needed. There is too often a tendency in hospitals to talk bracingly to patients, since few physicians and nurses are trained to listen. The ability to listen sympathetically appears to be rare. One of the most important functions of the staff is to encourage children and their parents to express feelings freely.

Many professionals in this field are too adult-centered and do not listen enough to what children say. Thus, they deprive themselves of the most potent diagnostic and therapeutic tools. These professionals tend to avoid anything that seems to resemble probing, for fear of further upsetting children. Facing feelings is more likely to help children come to terms with them. The urge to re-assure children by minimizing worries and by promising speedy recovery generally stems from the natural, but mistaken, assumption that they would lose control and become frightened if their anxieties were taken seriously. Faced with their own anxieties about the children's emotional distress, many workers shut off defensively when a painful topic is raised by a child. Hospital personnel often maintain that the current quick turnover in pediatric wards allows little time to attend to and explore children's feelings and thoughts. The observations of members of our study groups on the effect of illness and hospitalization, however, have shown abundantly that hospitalized children can respond to a person who gives attention. It is possible to gain important insights even during very short contacts if children are not distracted by reassurances and attempts to jolly them out of distress. Even very young and relatively inarticulate children will convey what is occupying them.

PERCEPTIONS OF PROCEDURES

We have learned about some specific reactions to the experience of illness and hospitalization including those of bewilderment, shock, anxiety, protest, withdrawal, indifference, compliance, or apparent acceptance. It will not take long, even for acutely ill or dying children, to go beyond these initial reactions to reveal the meaning of the experience to the skilled observer. It is this intimate, personal knowledge of individual children that will enable those taking care of them to be understanding and truly supportive.

Children often convey their fear of having been abandoned by their parents. They think they have been left to the mercy of strangers who might hurt or damage them. One of the hardest problems for children to face is how to adjust to being ill while brothers and sisters are well and at home with the parents. Frequently, illness and confinement in hospital are perceived as a punishment for a real or imagined undiscovered act of wrongdoing. The symbolic meaning of confinement then weighs more heavily than the actual act of wrongdoing and its consequences. By the same token, children may fear that other, perhaps worse, misdeeds will yet be discovered and dealt with similarly in the future. Whether these fears relate to real or fantasied activities appears to make little difference to children's interpretation of illness as being deserved punishment. When in the grip of such thoughts they cannot perceive reality objectively; they will put it in the service of the fantasy and wonder why doctors and nurses, who are supposed to make them feel better, subject them to procedures such as taking blood, giving injections and lumbar punctures, and requiring nasty-tasting medicines. Operations pose a great worry to children who may perceive them as some sort of mutilation or annihilation. Certainly circumcision, unless it is performed very early in infancy, tends to be considered a punishment. Hospitalization and, in the case of an infectious disease, isolation add to the fear of being rejected, expelled, unloved, and unlovable. It is important for hospital staff to take into account the children's perceptions of such procedures as being attacks on them by a hostile environment.

Diets, too, can be seen as serious deprivations. They are intolerable since, because of the satisfaction of early oral needs, children equate food with love.

In addition, young children are particularly frightened of any type of interference with bodily openings. They strongly resist suppositories, enemas, catheterization, or examinations of ears and eyes. There is much clinical evidence to suggest that these interventions are seen as invasions or seductions. These interventions mobilize children's anxieties and attendant defensive reactions.

Painful procedures of all kinds are apt to arouse and make manifest children's latent masochistic tendencies. We also know that medical investigations are feared by many children because they experience these as an intrusive scrutiny of the body that may reveal hidden secrets. This anxiety is often the result of fear arising from sexual fantasies and masturbation that they worry has caused damage to their bodies.

Clinical experience has also taught us that surgical intervention or any kind of interference with the body is likely to arouse fantasies and fears of being hurt, attacked, damaged, mutilated, or deprived of valuable parts of the body. Hence, some children want to keep whatever was removed by surgery, including their stitches. They seem to treasure them. For some, these visible trophies of their sufferings are then displayed proudly to others. When encouraged postoperatively to express thoughts and concerns, children frequently express the fear that the operation scar might open. For this reason, the very suggestion that stitches will be removed terrifies them. A procedure such as shaving hair from the head before neurosurgery can be a most disconcerting experience for children. It leaves the head exposed and unprotected. The suggestion that a beautiful wig can be chosen may fail to be either amusing or comforting.

For the same reasons, tests can cause a great deal of anxiety, especially if their purpose is not understood or if they have caused physical discomforts. The mysteries of making a diagnosis are difficult for children. They experience relief when they are able to assign a name to the illness. It makes scarcely any difference to the children whether the intervention is, by objective standards, a minor or a major one. These implications should be fully understood because staff and parents are naturally very concerned with and influenced by the severity of the intervention. Consequently they may respond sympathetically to the distress of children who have faced major procedures but may show little empathy or concern for one who has been exposed to a relatively minor treatment or surgery.

In the strange and often frightening environment of the hospital, with all the attendant pain and anxiety to be borne, the children attach a special value to their beds; this is the only place that is their own, and that they associate with warmth and comfort. The bed is home and should be allowed to remain the children's place of refuge and security. Therefore, unpleasant, painful procedures should never, if at all avoidable, be carried out in the child's bed.

A greater understanding of the discrepancies between children's psychic and physical reality would decrease the exasperation of the hospital staff and greatly reduce distress among child patients.

THE EMOTIONAL NEEDS OF PARENTS

As parents know too well, at home sick children do not always play during the acute stage of illness but only when they begin to get better. In the hospital, there is the danger that play and play specialists are being used to lull the staff into the comforting belief that a child is fully taken care of just because he is kept occupied and temporarily distracted from pain, discomfort, and anxieties. It is unfortunately fashionable in some quarters in England to look upon play as a panacea, attributing to it almost automatic and magical benefits that it clearly does not have. Although this belief springs from a desire to create a friendly atmosphere on the ward, it may deceptively lead the staff to believe that they are caring for all the emotional needs of the children. This is not so. The complexity of sick children's emotional states requires that good care must also include attention to the emotional needs of the family. Children's ability to cope with illness and hospitalization can be strengthened or undermined by the quality of the support that the parents give. In turn, the parents' ability to perform a supporting role will frequently depend on the understanding of professionals. Parents need to feel confident that the hospital staff are willing and able to help them and that they will be treated with honesty and respect.

Parents have as much need as the child of sustained emotional support. Staff should listen to them sympathetically and encourage them to express their concerns freely. When there is friction between parents and staff, it can usually be traced to a lack of regular and honest communication. The most common complaint from parents about doctors is that "they never tell you anything" or "you have to fight to get information." The staff frequently answer this accusation by maintaining that the parents did not pay attention to what was told to them and that great care had been taken to give the information. The staff sometimes complain that parents' anxious behavior upsets the children and that parents generally make nuisances of themselves.

When parents become labeled as difficult or overanxious, the staff may need help to grasp the fact that parents need as much sympathetic understanding as their child. Under severe emotional stress, parents worry about their child's condition, the possible complications and aftereffects, and responsibility for treatment. Parents may also suffer a sense of guilt about the origin of the disease, perhaps even feeling responsible for it. Given such emotional turmoil, they naturally find it hard to absorb what they are told by the staff. Far from being too stupid or incompetent to follow instructions or, as has been suggested occasionally, deliberately obstructive, they are more likely to be too emotionally preoccupied with their own fears and anxieties to give their full attention to what is said to them. It is important for those whose responsibility it is to talk to parents to remember that, in addition to giving information honestly and carefully, they must also be ready and willing to listen to parents' worries. They must repeat the information many times to insure that the facts are correctly understood and that their implications are absorbed.

Equally, when the child leaves hospital, those who will take over the responsibility for aftercare, such as the family doctor or public health nurse, need to have full information about the case. This type of follow-up is essential in instances of chronic illness that require fixed routines and diets. Children who had been anxious to return home were frequently reluctant to leave the hospital because they were worried about how they would be able to manage at home. These children worried whether their families would be competent to deal with their condition. This is especially true in the case of a continuing handicap. Children ask, "Who would know how to look after me or when to give me my injections?" and "What can I eat?" They are afraid to leave the hospital that, for all its strangeness, did at least understand the illness.

Children whose mothers have had a difficult time dealing with their own anxieties, or whose mothers are very excitable, often present a special problem. These mothers tend to lack confidence in their own ability to deal with the illness. We know of children who have had to bear the whole burden of their own illness unsupported, battling with experiences that would baffle even adults. This burden was clearly too much for them to cope with.

How and by whom can the needs of the sick child and his family be met? To begin with, all members of the pediatric team can make their contribution through understanding and sympathetic behavior in the everyday contact with the child. What is most clearly required, however, is a worker whose main function is to act as an intermediary between the child's family and the hospital.

TRAINING FOR STAFF

When the hospital staff take on a supporting role, they need continuing help and encouragement. Psychological training should be available to them as well as consultation on the day-to-day problems of child patients and their families. At present such training is lacking in the majority of our medical and nursing schools where, for some rather extraordinary reason, it is still widely assumed that skills concerning human relations develop on their own. It follows, therefore, that those who will be selected for training in this field will be men and women with a natural capacity for compassion. Training in casework techniques and interviewing skills adds to the understanding of the roots and meanings of anxieties.

Pediatricians are increasingly asked to expand their sphere beyond its traditional limits of diagnosing and treating physical illness. It is becoming more widely understood that psychology is as necessary to effective maintenance of children's health as is knowledge of physical disease. The physician who maintains the medical side of his role cannot, however, as Dr. Donald Winnicott put it, "slip quietly over to child psychiatry." The terms, techniques and concepts of dynamic psychology, though familiar, are part of a new science, one that is not found in the basic curriculum of the medical student or the student nurse.

The specialist's task is not only to help children directly but also to help the staff to understand the complexity of children's mental and emotional functioning. Efforts to promote such understanding among all people concerned with the care of children is essential for the promotion of better patient-staff relationships. Clearly, before the hospital staff can develop an approach to embrace the welfare of the whole child, they must come to respect the position and point of view of child psychiatry and be guided to an understanding of the principles of work in psychology.

Total care, which recognizes the interdependence of physical and psychological factors, is an essential prerequisite for what must surely be one of the most urgent objectives: the cure not only of the illness itself but also of the whole person of the child, thus preventing subsequent damage to the child's emotional health. Theoretical knowledge alone is not enough to equip a worker for the kind of task that I have described. The ability to perform well depends to a large degree on the personality of the professional who cares for sick children and their parents. In specific terms, what is needed is the ability to empathize and to form a relationship with patients. This ability is based not on the acceptance of theoretical guidelines, so vehemently sought by some professionals, but rather on genuine compassion. Without compassion words and actions have a hollow ring. These personal qualities can be found in any personnel. Patients and families, giving accounts of the hospital experience, have singled out hospital porters, ward orderlies, student nurses, and medical students as examples of understanding contacts in an otherwise impersonal hospital setting. The approach that is appreciated is a spontaneous, natural reaction by one human being to another, a warmth toward people in distress, an acceptance of others as equals, empathy, and an untiring willingness to help. Compassion seems to be the most important attribute.

The qualities of kindness and compassion are, of course, essential, but they are not sufficient on their own for the ideal balance of competent physical and psychological care of children in hospital. Staff need deeper and more specific knowledge so that they can be of greater help to the child patient and can make better use of limited resources. This brings us to look at demands for further intensive theoretical research into the emotional needs of sick children and their families.

NEED FOR RESEARCH

Although I welcome research into areas in which we need to break new ground, I question the need for further studies into aspects about which considerable knowledge has been available for quite a long time. Our day-to-day work offers us excellent opportunities to explore the needs of children. By asking children and their parents about their feelings and attitudes, about what they find helpful or otherwise, and by showing interest in their replies in a way that invites honest statements, we are afforded the best possible chance for research. Thus, we can enrich our knowledge not only about individual needs but also about the effectiveness of the services we are trying to provide.

I strongly feel that we need to study the reasons for our failure to develop services that make use of the knowledge we already possess about the emotional aspects of sickness and hospitalization. The hospital, more than any other institution, offers a unique opportunity for identifying and treating emotional stress. The consequences of such stress can be easily anticipated in the hospital, whether it relates to the birth of a baby, to an illness, to an injury, or to a death in the family. In the hospital immediate efforts to alleviate the consequences of stressful experiences can be made.

The beneficial effects of preventive work more than justify the concerted efforts in training and management. This work not only relieves present suffering but also obviates protracted and expensive treatment at a later stage. To this end all those who work with sick children should combine their efforts. These practical opportunities for unified interdisciplinary action among specialists can produce a working climate in which theory and practice are not separated. None of us and not one of our professions can tackle alone the problem of sick children and the needs of their families. Together we must strive to translate existing knowledge into effective action.

SUMMARY

The reasons for our failure to achieve satisfactory standards of comprehensive care for children and their families can hardly be attributed to the lack of theoretical knowledge or to the lack of agreement about the way in which projected policies should be put into practice but rather to our hesitation to take the deliberate step from rational agreement to implementation.

Treatment should be based on the awareness of the child as a person whose body and mind are interrelated and inseparable. Treatment, therefore, requires interdisciplinary cooperation and not the isolated efforts of different departments and professional disciplines. Children must be treated as an integral part of their families. The families' needs and problems have a bearing on the children's physical and emotional recovery and are our concern and responsibility. Concerted practical action must be crystallized out of the crucible of theoretical knowledge. Although the change may be difficult initially, we are the catalysts who can make progress possible.

The child in the hospital bed who for so long has been a familiar stranger must no longer be able to say, "They looked into my mouth and into my ears; they looked into my eyes, and they touched my tummy, but they never looked at me."

2

singing: an aid to parental attachment

JOHN LIND

John Lind, MD, Professor Emeritus at Karolinska Institute in Stockholm, encourages expectant and new mothers to sing to their babies. This project, developed in Sweden and the United States, demonstrates a method in which communication and closeness can develop among mother, father, and baby.

Wherever there are people there is music. Despite variances from culture to culture each epoch has its music. There is music for daily enjoyment, for ceremonials and rituals, for prayer chants, for work songs, for songs of celebration, for play, and for grief. Throughout history, the binding force that makes music out of mere sounds is rhythm, and that rhythm is present even before birth.

The rhythmical throbbing of the mother's heart is one of the first stimuli received by the brain of the unborn child. The child senses the mother's rhythmical breathing and rhythmical stride as she walks. Life for the unborn child is accompanied by continuous, vibrating, pulsating, wavelike movement. The child developing in the dark chamber of the womb receives a constant stream of sensory stimuli. These impressions nourish the brain and encourage its growth.

It is probable that later in life sounds akin to heartbeats are associated, more or less consciously, with the memory of the heartbeat of the mother and that such sounds help the child feel secure by settting the reassuring rhythm of life(1).

Viewed in this light it is easy to understand the use of the word *heart* in situations connected with love and strong feelings of belonging. A parent calls the baby "my little sweetheart." We use terms of approval such as "her heart is in the right place" or "he's a good-hearted soul." These expressions indicate our perception of love as originating in the heart(1).

Certain patterns of human behavior indicate that we are correct in attaching such importance to the heart. For example, a study of the way in which mothers hold their infants found that eighty percent of the right-handed mothers held children on their left side near the heart(1). This might be explained by saying that it is the most comfortable and natural way for a right-handed person to hold a baby, but the same study indicated that left-handed mothers do the same thing. Furthermore, from the age of six, little girls tend to hold their dolls on the left side(2).

Perhaps this is instinctive behavior in girls and women. What sort of instinctive behavior do boys and men display regarding care of infants? Nobody knows the answer yet. Fathers have not been regarded as being quite as interesting to observe in their relationships to children as have mothers. You might say that fathers have been treated somewhat heartlessly.

An important medical discovery showed that the unborn child's hearing faculty develops during the fifth, sixth, and seventh months of pregnancy(3). During this period and up to approximately twelve months after birth, the size and inner structure of the child's brain is in a state of intensive growth. New nerve fibers shoot out, proliferate, and ramify. The fibers become linked together partly as a result of the stimuli of a stream of external impressions.

After the seventh month of pregnancy it is no longer only the heart of the mother that provides rhythmical and auditory stimuli. Her voice is also heard by the unborn child. Vibrating and strong, it penetrates the womb. It can be assumed that the unborn child learns to recognize this voice from the fact that, as early as the second day after birth, the newborn infant can recognize its own mother's voice. When the infant is held up and the mother stands behind so that the child cannot see her, the baby makes movements in the direction of the mother's voice. The infant is not interested in other voices(4).

Like the sound of her heartbeat, the mother's voice when she speaks or sings acts as a link with the child after the umbilical cord is severed. Her voice is a factor contributing to the child's feeling of security. Most parents know that they should sing, hum, or croon to their children right from birth, but perhaps we should sing to the baby even before birth. I am strongly inclined to think so. Pregnant mothers who enjoy listening to music and who sing and perform themselves notice that a nervous, jumpy baby calms down when music is sung or played. Some mothers say that if the music suddenly gets loud, the unborn baby startles. Loud music can wake the unborn child from slumber and cause it to start kicking even if the baby is not frightened by the sound, although not all kicking is caused by loud music.

When the mother- and father-to-be talk, sing, or play an instrument, it is important for them to imagine that they are addressing the unborn baby and to pay attention to the response. It is not uncommon for a mother to have difficulty realizing that the child is really hers even after the child is born. This feeling of alienation, an inability to get used to the idea of having her own child, may persist for quite a while. Some women become unhappy and depressed with a sense of failure, and they worry that the feeling of belonging together might not ever develop. Although this is generally an unfounded fear, I believe that by addressing the unborn child during the course of pregnancy that a mother can get acquainted with her baby. This attachment can heighten her sense of nurturing after the child is born. Singing to the baby before its birth is a way for her to get a head start on attachment. The mother can become aware of her infant's prenatal responses to her voice and to her rhythms; she can notice what is soothing and what is stimulating.

What would help the father to realize that he has a child? He, too, can begin communicating with the unborn child by listening to the baby's heart. Although the mother can do this only on those special occasions when she can borrow a stethoscope, the father can put his ear against the mother's abdomen and listen directly to the child's heart at about three months from the end of the pregnancy. When he listens directly to the child's heart, he can describe to the mother what he hears. These are the gestures and behaviors that encourage attachment and the realization of parenthood.

In other cultures, South America, Africa, and Asia, where these customs have been retained, the awaiting baby is regarded as an individual person and as a member of the family whose presence is real. In China, for instance, the age of the child is not reckoned from the moment of birth but from conception. They say it is one year old at birth. In Nepal the father-to-be sings to his unborn child. Sitting close to the mother, he improvises tunes and words that tell how impatiently they are all looking forward to the baby's arrival and describes all the wonderful things that life holds for the child.

A PARENT SINGING PROGRAM

In one of our Swedish maternity hospitals, we encouraged new parents to gather and sing lullabies(5). At first, there were many protests. "I can't sing." "I was terrible at music in school." "I was never allowed to sing in chorus." "I don't know any lullabies." Then a young woman with a guitar, who came in to lead the new parents in singing, gave them the words to some well-known lullabies. Little by little the singing got under way, and even those parents who preferred not to sing in the group took the lullaby song sheets home with them. They were assured that singing when they felt like singing would be a help to their child and a help to them. A suitable song for singing to infants, we told them, is any song one feels like singing. It could be an old song from one's own childhood. Perhaps it could be a special something that a parent wants to say to the baby, a melody made up as she goes along. New parents were advised:

> Everyone is born with a voice, and that is the voice to use. That is the voice that your child recognizes. So sing, father and mother. You, who have never dared to open your mouth to sing when anyone is around, can give it a go with your own baby. There is nothing to fear. No one is asking for a concert performance! Humming, crooning, croaking—in the eyes and ears of your child you have just the right voice. You have the only voice on this earth that has just the right effect on your child.

Music and rhythm bring joy to listener and musician alike and develop feelings of communion. The musical interplay between parent and child increases their sense of belonging to each other. In developing this communication they make use of a gift for which they have paid nothing, since music is a language inherited by us all. The experiences that we share when we sing, play instruments, or listen to each other become the cornerstones of a strong, stable foundation on which to build the family's future.

REFERENCES

1. Salk, L. The role of the heartbeat in the relationship between mother and infant. *Scientific American*, May 1973, *228*, 24–29.
2. Chateau, P. de. *Neonatal care routines: Influences on maternal and infant behaviour and on breast feeding.* Thesis, University of Umeå (Sweden), 1976.
3. Sontag, L. W., & Wallace, R. F. Changes in the rate of the human fetal heart in response to vibratory stimuli. *American Journal of Diseases of Children*, 1936, *51*, 583–589.
4. Hutt, S. J. Auditory discrimination at birth. In S. J. Hutt and C. Hutt (Eds.), *Early human development.* Oxford: Oxford University Press, 1973.
5. Lind, J., & Hardgrove, C. Lullabies. *Children Today*, 1978, *7*, 7–9.

3

family issues
in diabetes

CALVIN R. KING, JR.

Calvin R. King, Jr., PhD, is an Assistant Professor with the Department of Psychiatry and Behavioral Sciences of the Medical University of South Carolina in Charleston. He describes the significant effects of family interactions on the course of the child's illness.

The emergence of psychological problems at the onset and during the subsequent course of juvenile diabetes is a frequently recognized clinical phenomenon. This lifelong and potentially life-threatening disease with its many difficulties places substantial levels of stress on the adaptive capacity of both child and parents. In addition, the day-in, day-out management of the disease presents further avenues for the expression of psychosocial conflicts within the child and the parents and between them. Thus, the psychological ramifications of juvenile diabetes become factors of considerable importance in the care of the child.

Health care staff, especially nursing staff, pediatricians, and dietitians, are often the first people to encounter the psychological reactions of the newly diagnosed child with diabetes and the child's parents. Similarly, the staff for the outpatient clinic following the child with diabetes as well as the staff of the inpatient metabolic unit may be in the most advantageous location to observe the longitudinal process of adaptation of both the child and the parents to the realities of the disease and its management. I will consider several different aspects in my discussion, especially the interactional significance of parent-child relationships relative to the special circumstances of the child with diabetes.

THE FAMILY'S ROLE IN TREATMENT

Three goals in the treatment of diabetes so that the child may achieve normal social functioning are(1): (a) maintaining the clinical control of the diabetic condition at a high level; (b) shifting the responsibility for care from the professional team to the parent and ultimately to the child; and (c) assisting the child and family in developing and maintaining a comfortable attitude toward the condition.

A common observation is that psychological stresses may promote hyperglycemia. If the distress is acute, an episode of ketoacidosis may be precipitated with associated complications. If the stress is chronic enough, it is conceivable that it may intensify the severity of the diabetic state. But psychosocial dysfunction may also affect the disease process, particularly by its influence on the personal health care behavior of the child. In most situations the appropriateness of the child's and family's behavior in relation to the diabetic treatment is directly proportional to the adequacy of patient education on good diabetic care. However, if the child has significant emotional and interpersonal problems there will likely be irregularities in urine monitoring, insulin preparation and injection, diet and exercise.

More than any other party, the parents' reaction can critically influence the impact the diabetes has on the psychological welfare of their child. By and large, if the parents adapt well, face the realities of the disease, accept their role in the management of treatment, and constructively cope with their emotional reactions, the child is more likely to adapt well, too. However, if the parents maladapt to the disease and its implications in any of several ways, for example by failing to recognize and learn about their role in treatment, or by catering to every whim of their child, the child is less likely to adapt well to the diabetes or even to typical developmental tasks.

Parental acceptance and constructive parental coping have been found to relate to good control(2). It is likely that these factors relate through multiple means. The child probably experiences less psychological distress if the parents are handling their feelings and their behaviors appropriately. Some children are prone to assume the burden of their parents' feelings and guilt, so it follows that the better the parents cope the less likely this phenomenon will occur.

Family adjustments are a critical factor. The family therapist, Minuchen(3), described a quite dramatic improvement in a group of labile children with diabetes whose families participated in family therapy. In addition, the expression of feelings by parents, particularly at the time of initial hospitalization, has been shown to occur more frequently among parents of well-controlled children than of poorly-controlled children(4). Apparently the ability to express feelings allows some parents to cope more effectively with the affects generated by the child's disease. I suspect, though, that there is a potential problem with that particular factor. We have seen parents who are quite expressive of their feelings at the time of diagnosis as well as later on, but who do not seem to use that awareness constructively. Their feelings continue to interfere and the continuing high levels of anxiety or emotionality may be transmitted to the child. The child may then maintain a heightened state of emotionality.

It is normal for parents to react intensely when suddenly confronted with a diagnosis of serious illness in their child. The problems begin when the parents' intense reactions become prolonged and they do not seem able to start dealing with the realities of the disease. The sooner the parents accept the disease, the sooner they can get about the business of realistic management. Although it is certainly difficult to have a child with a chronic illness, I have observed some parents who became so caught up in their own emotional reactions to the child's diagnosis that they seem to have lost sight of who the patient really is.

DEVELOPMENTAL FRAMEWORK FOR BEHAVIOR

I would like to look now at a conceptual framework that provides knowledge of normal ranges of behavior during various stages of development. That knowledge may help families and staff to anticipate and evaluate the emotional and behavioral reactions of the child not only at the time of diagnosis but also throughout the child's development.

Juvenile onset diabetes, unlike some other medical problems that may arise in childhood, requires treatment from the moment of diagnosis onward. There is no let-up; it goes on throughout the life of the patient. Thus there can be no temporary suspension of treatment to wait until a more opportune moment in development for intervention. For the child with diabetes, treatment must proceed regardless of what other psychological issues may be of importance at that particular time. I bring this out because of some other conditions that may arise, for example, with the child requiring elective surgery, it may be possible to delay medical intervention until the child is developmentally better able to cope with that stress. From early infancy through preschool years, the child with diabetes is virtually a victim of the disease and unable to understand what is happening. The infant with diabetes may be aware only of the painful stimulation from insulin injections. If the infant is overwhelmed by excessive painful stimulation, that experience may serve as a prototype for psychic helplessness that may then set the tone for heightened levels of psychological vulnerability later on.

The parents are the only buffer for the infant and the young child. McArthur(5) noted that the "Parents are in a crucial position to modulate the effect that the illness has on the psychological life of the child." The crucial variable may be the parents' affective response to the child's illness. Erikson(6) has said that a child and even a baby sensitively reflect the quality of the milieu in which they grow up. Children feel the tensions, insecurities, and rages of their parents even if they do not know their causes or witness their more overt manifestations. Thus the parents' feelings about the child's illness may be conveyed to the child and the child may express tension, fearfulness, or sadness.

Another factor during very early years of childhood is that of separation. During the second year of life the mother is gradually perceived as existing apart from the child. Yet at the same time she is considered by the child with increasing importance; the mother's absence, therefore, becomes frightening and dangerous to the child, who may experience the separation as abandor.ment. Hospitals increasingly provide the opportunity for parents to remain with their child.

The principal developmental task of the toddler phase is that of separation-individuation in which the child goes about the work of establishing a psychological and physical separation from the parents, beginning to work on the task of establishing a sense of individuality. During this phase of development the child can become quite oppositional. Control battles may emerge between parent and child that tax the parents' composure. For the child with diabetes and the parents this can become a particularly trying time. The parents must continue to administer the diabetic treatment regardless of possible active opposition by a child who still may not understand why this is all necessary. At the same time the parents must continue to show the child affection, nurturance, and love despite strained relations. A critical danger at this stage is the child's loss of esteem if parental love is withdrawn in the face of the child's opposition.

As the child's development passes on to the preschool years new developmental tasks emerge and older ones are refined. The child is becoming more independent and more of a social person. Peer activities and play with or without the presence of another child occupy a good part of the day. For the child with diabetes it is important to support participation in play and peer activities, so the child will not see himself as being greatly different from his peers, a fact that investigators have noted for some time in children with physical disabilities. From this point on throughout

childhood and adolescence the importance of peer group participation cannot be overestimated.

A danger that psychoanalysts note during this particular
stage of development is that of the child's fear of damage or injury to the body. As the child gradually develops and emerges as
a person separate and apart from the parents and develops a perception of his own body integrity, it is conceivable that the neces-
sity of daily injections of insulin will elicit greater fear from the
child at this time than at other times in development.

The child is also involved in the process of identification.
When a diabetic child has a parent who has diabetes, the attitudes
and behaviors of the parent may serve as a model for attitudes and
behaviors in the child. One diabetic child, who was hospitalized in
the psychiatric unit, had a diabetic father. The father did not take
care of himself, he ate what he wanted when he wanted to. In
anticipation of his food intake, the father would increase the
dosage of insulin and was generally irresponsible about his care.
Obviously the child did not have an appropriate model within
his family for proper care of diabetes. It was extremely difficult for
the child to cope adequately and to use the information that he
had to take care of himself.

In the elementary school years much of the child's energy is
directed towards the mastery of a variety of tasks. The tasks include the acquisition of knowledge in and outside of school, the
mastery of a variety of physical skills, and the development of social skills. Much importance is attached to peer relationships. The
esteem and regard with which the child views himself is dependent
in large part on the child's perception of his own capabilities and
of his perception of doing well in social, physical, and intellectual
tasks. Given this emphasis on achievement in latency, it would
seem theoretically sound for the child who has diabetes to be encouraged during this particular stage of development to begin the
mastery of those tasks that are essential for the control of the
disease. The degree of the mastery would depend on the task to
be accomplished as well as on several other factors. For example,
meeting the dietary requirements of the disease, usually carried
out within the context of the family's eating habits with food
typically prepared by the parent, may not be realistically mastered
until well into adolescence. Yet, it is both conceivable and em-

pirically sound that the latency stage child can acquire sufficient knowledge of the dietary requirements to help with meal planning and occasionally to prepare a meal without adult supervision. Other tasks may be mastered in their entirety during this period; for example, the injections of insulin may be accomplished at a fairly young age. A pediatric diabetologist who has been the physician at a camp for children with diabetes reported that children as young as six years of age are measuring and administering their own insulin. These children are usually under the supervision of the parents, but they are quite able to do it themselves if needed.

RESOURCES FOR THE FAMILY

The American Diabetes Association and the Juvenile Diabetes Foundation, two organizations that provide a great deal of education, information, and research activities in the area of diabetes, provide an important function through the local affiliates as one type of support for parents and children. For many families this may be their primary source of emotional and social support. Occasionally, some parents become overcommitted and use organizational participation as a means of expressing great concern for the welfare of the child, almost as a defensive way of avoiding the nitty-gritty task of dealing with the child or with their own feelings, thoughts, and conflicts about the diabetes. For example, I have seen a parent become very interested in trying to get publicity in the newspapers or on television about juvenile diabetes and the particular kinds of problems involved. Such parents have to be warned that they may create emotional troubles by getting their child in front of the television camera to tell what it is like to live with diabetes. In this particular instance the child did not want to do it and told the parents so. Fortunately the parents backed off, but it is that sort of overly-committed parent who concerns me.

COMMENT: You were describing overly-committed behavior as a defense against anxiety. I think that is quite true for some.

Another explanation, however, which is not all that uncommon, is that there are people who like to have their child sick, for various reasons. There are mothers who, if they have a child with diabetes, feel that at last someone needs them.

KING: Yes, that happens. And it emphasizes the need for consultation for mental health services. This could be detected either during the child's initial hospitalization or during follow-up visits or subsequent hospitalizations. Such services can be offered when the pediatrician or nurse or anyone else working with the child gains the impression that emotional conflicts are interfering with the proper management or with the process of coping with normal development. One approach(7) to consultation is based on the premise that emotional dysfunction involves an inability to express affect both freely and in a reasonable manner. A crisis such as the diagnosis of diabetes, with all its ramifications, may generate a powerful affect and overtax the ability of the child and the parents to deal with it. When this occurs it is suggested that the pediatrician should empathically confront the child rather than avoid the child's feelings by reasoning or other intellectualized approaches. Psychiatric consultation is suggested in the following circumstances: (a) when reasonable confrontation alone does not make the child aware of affect; (b) when the child or family is aware of affect but is unable to express it other than through maladaptive means; (c) when internalized emotional conflicts repeatedly generate painful affect in a child.

More typically the psychiatrist or psychologist consults on dealing with the here-and-now kinds of problems that emerge on the pediatric service.

Groups can also operate in a hospital to meet the emotional needs of parents. At the hospital where I work there is an ongoing group that has an open- or revolving-door policy for parents of children who are hospitalized for any reason. The group provides a trained leader and an opportunity for the parents to begin dealing with the feelings that the child's hospitalization has generated. Therapy groups have also been recommended for dealing with adolescent patients. Another treatment possibility is structural family therapy(8), an approach that focuses on three interrelated areas of the family unit: the first focuses on the way the family functions; the second focuses on what is referred to as the ecosystem, including the whole community, school, church, and peers; and the third focuses on the developmental level of the family.

These various approaches to the psychological problems that emerge in the treatment of the child who has diabetes can be helpful interventions and can assist in the control of the disease.

REFERENCES

1. Garner, A. M., & Thompson, C. W. Juvenile diabetes. In P. R. Magrab (Ed.), *Psychological management of pediatric problems. Vol. 1: Early life conditions and chronic disease.* Baltimore: University Park Press, 1978.
2. Koski, M. L. The coping processes in childhood diabetes. *Acta Paediatrica Scandinavica,* Suppl. 198, 1969.
3. Minuchin, S.; Baker, L.; Rosman, B. L.; Liebman, R.; Milman, L., & Todd, T. C. A conceptual model of psychosomatic illness in children: Family organization and family therapy. *Archives of General Psychiatry,* 1975, *32,* 1031–1038.
4. Koski, op. cit.
5. McArthur, R. G., Tomm, K. M., & Leahey, M. D. Management of diabetes mellitus in children. *Canadian Medical Association Journal,* 1976, *114,* 783–787.
6. Erickson, E. H. Growth and crises of the healthy personality. *Psychological Issues,* 1959, *1,* 50–100.
7. Carek, D. J. Focus on affect: The pediatrician and empathic confrontation. *Clinical Pediatrics,* 1978, *17,* 547–578.
8. Hodas, G. R., & Liebman, R. Psychosomatic disorders in children: Structural family therapy. *Psychosomatics,* 1978, *19,* 709–719.

4

the impact
of end-stage
renal disease

BARBARA KORSCH

Barbara Korsch, MD, Professor of Pediatrics in the School of Medicine, University of Southern California, Los Angeles, describes the effects of emotional care on the survival of seriously ill children.

We have been involved for twelve years in treating children with end-stage renal disease at Childrens Hospital of Los Angeles. We have done 250 kidney transplants on children, and we run a dialysis program for children while they are awaiting transplantation. From the beginning of the program it was clear that this was going to be a devastating experience for children and their families and that we should be very conscientious about documenting what this treatment did to the children, to the families, and to the staff. There were those who felt in those days, and some who still feel, that the cost of this kind of treatment program for children, not only in terms of individual and community dollars, but also in terms of human suffering for the child and family, might be too great to warrant prolonging lives of children with end-stage renal disease. We felt the only way to answer that question would be to gather data conscientiously as we went along, a systematic, psychosocial follow-up study, and to try to learn what it really did mean to all concerned and what we could do to help them through the experience.

The emphasis has been to determine whether there are some specific stresses involved in the treatment of this disease that are different from other chronic illnesses. We all know that any major catastrophic illness is a stressful experience and that many of the manifestations in the children and families that we observed are nonspecific stress reactions. Some stress reactions are common to all chronic illnesses, but we were curious to know if there was anything special that we could learn about this particular experience that would help us help the patients better. We had to learn when to give anticipatory guidance to patients and families, since there are ups and downs through the various phases of illness, dependency on the machine, and all the implications of receiving an organ transplant. We found moments when we had to get children together with other children to prepare them for experiences. There were other times when the parents needed special support.

Our interdisciplinary psychosocial team began to do simple assessments of the family and child in a systematic fashion. Many of the instruments we used were chosen so that we could compare our families with families of other children. We did a family intake, for example, that is fashioned after that used in some other studies. Our intake/interview included a series of simple pen-and-paper personality tests. One of our criteria for selecting tests was to have something that would not require a team of psychiatrists, psychologists, or other people trained at great length, and that would not take too much time. We hoped that we would come up with data that the ordinary health care providers might be able to incorporate in their assessments of children. We have not done extensive projective tests or in-depth psychiatric interviews except when they were clinically indicated. We have tried to use tests that are readily administered, readily interpreted, and useful.

The personality tests we used were surprisingly informative. We used the California Test of Personality(1), for example. We chose it because it could be applied to many age groups, and our patient population ranges from infancy through late adolescence. We also chose it because it had been successfully used and standardized on thousands of children in the school system, and it was easy to score and administer. It has been singularly helpful. People can hardly believe that it tells you so much, since the questions are very simple.

We also gave the Piers-Harris Self-Esteem Test(2). It had been well-standardized and used by the Rochester group. We certainly feel, as I am sure you do, that self-esteem is one of the aspects of personality function that is most likely to suffer with chronic illness of this kind. Also, there is a good deal of evidence that suggests that self-esteem has a very good predictive value in terms of rehabilitation and patients' health behavior.

We have done various tests of anxiety and up to now we have never found one to be useful over a great many age groups. What makes a very young child anxious may be perfectly normal for that age, like being afraid of the dark, but would be unusual in an adolescent. Finally, we used a draw-a-person test to see what happened to their image of themselves. We also asked them to draw what is inside the human body. We used developmental intelligence tests when they were indicated, not as part of the profile. We have data on 150 patients who have been followed from one to twelve years of age. In general, our results have been very encouraging.

ADAPTIVE AND MALADAPTIVE BEHAVIOR

Within one year after transplantation, children reentered school at an appropriate level and renewed their social and family life. If there were preexisting problems, obviously transplantation and treatment for end-stage renal disease would not change that. To the extent that these young people have returned to expected activity levels of rehabilitation, we have had very gratifying results. Eleven of our transplant patients, of which two are male, have offspring. The women have delivered babies normally and I have taken care of most of those babies. We have not had any congenital anomalies, and we have no reason to think they cannot go through normal childbearing. There are some complications and we have published those (3, 4). In the overall sample, an appropriate number are married and an appropriate number have jobs, so with our overall kind of rehabilitation data we are very pleased.

I do want to talk to you about various kinds of maladaptations in these patients, however, and the importance of providing psychosocial support. We have found that some children will go through the whole experience with end-stage renal disease, the hemodialysis and transplantation, and will have a functioning kidney. Then, as those of you who work with this kind of patient know, the children have to take two kinds of medication to keep the body from rejecting the kidney. One of them is Imuran and the other one is some form of corticosteroid. We have had a significant percent of patients who, after a period of time, will stop taking their immunosuppressive medication and will thereby either cause damage to their kidney or lose their graft. This is a tremendous loss to the child and the family and a terrible blow to the treatment team, as well as a great expense to the community. We have attempted to determine what would make a young person, who had gone through this horrendous experience and had the functioning kidney transplant, fail to take the medications. At first we thought it was simply because of the undesirable side effects, but this has not proven to be true.

We came across this phenomenon because gradually, clinically, we would find some of the children were noncompliant. It is interesting that it is usually a member of the psychosocial team, not one of the physicians, who learns about the noncompliance. It is very hard for a patient to go to the doctor who prescribed the medicine and say, "I have not been taking it," but they will tell the public health nurse or the social worker.

When we were analyzing our data on the personality tests we

made a table just of those children who have the lowest results on the personality tests. We found that a very high percent of our noncompliant patients were in this group. By viewing these simple personality tests we found we could identify some of the children who were likely to have serious trouble, such as noncompliance.

We have since done studies (5) to attempt to categorize those patients and families that are at a very high risk for maladaptation. We would like to be able to predict noncompliance, for example. We are now running a protocol because we found that when we isolated certain items from the personality tests and certain items from the family function, we could put together a formula for a computer to select the noncompliant patients. We are currently engaged in this predictive study and are attempting to see whether with various kinds of intervention we are perhaps able to break this very discouraging cycle. It is discouraging that, in spite of our maximum intervention and in spite of predicting some of the children who are likely to maladapt, our success with intervention has not been very great. Our current feeling is that if we have a patient who comes to the program with a vulnerable personality structure and who has little support from the family, a family in which there are poor communication patterns, the patient has a high risk for problems. The amount and timing of the intervention that we use in the course of their treatment program is just too little and too late.

The first few patients we had observed were adolescent girls who mind terribly about the way they look with steroids. One or two of them told us, "If I'm going to look like that, no. I wish I had not started the whole treatment program; I don't want to go back to high school looking like that," even though we had assured them that these are temporary effects. But the cause of noncompliance did not turn out to be as simple as dislike of undesirable side effects. It seems that those children and young people who grossly maladapt to our program tend to be those who come from a poorly communicating, not very supportive family, who themselves have already had personality damage. There is also a high risk, especially for noncompliance, in the adolescent female. The boys seem to show other kinds of maladaptation, but noncompliance with the immunosuppressant medication is most common in the adolescent female. So, if you take a vulnerable female adolescent and put her through this kind of experience, the probability of her getting through it intact seems poor. Out of six female adolescent patients who lost a kidney because of not taking medicine, who then were put back on dialysis, and who were given another kidney, three did not comply the second time and lost their second kidney.

All kinds of philosophic problems are raised that my colleagues may want to take up. There are some people, for instance, who feel that if a patient has not complied with the first kidney, we should not put the patient back on hemodialysis or give another one. I, for one, feel that capital punishment would be a severe response to noncompliance and that it would be ridiculous not to offer treatment programs with maximal support. But I must confess to you, sadly, that so far our results with the kind of interventions we have been able to mount, even with a fairly complex psychosocial support team, have not been that successful. I hate to end on a negative note, and I know those of you who visit us will attest to the fact that we do have, in general, a very active, cheerful, comprehensive program with many good results, but I thought for your interest I would present these problem areas.

REFERENCES

1. Thorpe, L. P., Clark, W. W., & Tiegs, E. W. *Manual, the California test of personality.* Monterey, CA: McGraw-Hill, 1953.
2. Piers, A. V., & Harris, D. B. Age and other correlates of self-concept. *Journal of Educational Psychology,* 1964, *55,* 91–95.
3. Korsch, B. M., Negrete, V. F., Gardner, J. E. et al. Kidney transplantation in children: Psychosocial follow-up study on child and family. *Journal of Pediatrics,* 1973, *83,* 399–408.
4. Korsch, B. M., Fine, R. N., & Negrete, V. F. Noncompliance in children with renal transplants. *Pediatrics,* 1978, *61,* 872–876.
5. Korsch, B. M., Klein, J. D., Negrete, V. F. et al. Physical and psychological follow-up on offspring of renal allograft recipients. *Pediatrics,* 180, *65,* 275.

5

family adaptation
after the death
of a child

JANET PAYNE

Janet Payne, ACSW, now at Tennessee's Department of Mental Health and Mental Retardation in Memphis, summarizes an effort to understand the psychosocial adjustment of families whose children died of cancer. This study was completed when she was a social worker at St. Jude Children's Research Hospital in Memphis.

Some children do die of cancer, despite the excellent treatment available today. Although we can focus on the quality of life of those who survive, we must not forget the families of those who do not. Because we wanted to know how families were coping after their child's death our hospital decided to study the effects of that traumatic event on the surviving family.

We wanted to know how the families who came to St. Jude were coping after their child died and what they thought about the treatment their child received.

Several similar studies have been done. A group(1) at the University of California, San Francisco Medical Center found that fifty-two percent of the families who lost a child to leukemia had one or more members who needed psychiatric help. A group(2) at Stanford University found that only twelve percent of the families studied were problem-free after they lost their child. A University of Iowa study(3) found that parents who lost a child reported a variety of symptoms such as loss of appetite, loss of weight, and preoccupation with thinking about their child, but they were free of these symptoms within six months. There are other studies, but let it suffice to say that it is known that families have significant problems for some time, since the loss of a child can be the most distressing of all griefs.

Most of the families who come to St. Jude are from out of town, so they are housed in several motels. For this reason, we usually see just the mother and the child since the father and the siblings are at home. You need to keep that in mind in thinking about the family unit.

To begin our study, we wrote letters to ninety-five families within a 100-mile radius and, in essence, said, "We would like to talk with you. What you say is confidential, but we are concerned." Eight letters were returned undeliverable, thirty-four parents wrote back and agreed to be interviewed but nine of these later changed their minds. Of the remaining twenty-five families, sixteen had lost a child within six months of our letter and nine families had lost a child within two years of our letter.

In eight of the six-month families and six of the two-year families data were collected on both parents. All of them were interviewed in their homes and each two-hour interview was taped.

Fifty-five percent of the six-month, and seventy-eight percent of the two-year families had incomes of over $10,000 a year. There were an equal number of rural and urban families. The mothers and fathers were somewhat older than we had expected and the majority of the parents were well educated, in that the mean of our population was a high school education.

The average age of the child who had died six months prior was twelve-and-a-half years; for those who had died two years earlier the average age was thirteen-and-a-half years. Eight of the children who had died six months previously had leukemia; six of those who died two years previously had leukemia. The other categories were aplastic anemia, muscular dystrophy, nonspecific diagnosis, and hemangiometosis. None of the children from the two-year group died at home whereas in the six-month group five of the children did so. I think this represents the current emphasis on families choosing to be with loved ones at home instead of in the hospital at the time of death.

In trying to decide how our parents coped we used a model(4) that indicates that grief progresses in four stages. The first phase is alarm, when people feel numb; this can last a few minutes to a couple of days. The second phase is a type of searching, looking for the deceased, being preoccupied with thoughts of him or her, and feeling guilty. The third phase is mitigation, when a person feels that the deceased is nearby, has a clear visual memory and begins to feel less sad. This is not to say that there is total adjustment to the loss, but rather that the loss becomes a part of the grieving person. The last stage is gaining a new identity, when functioning begins again in such a way that the person is no longer preoccupied with the deceased but has incorporated the loss.

We found the following to be significant in our six-month and two-year families: the six-month families reported feeling panicky, having headaches, and crying, to a significant degree, whereas our two-year families were experiencing predominantly two of the thirty-four symptoms that we looked at, that is, feeling guilty and feeling angry.

We asked what the parents did with the belongings of their deceased child. Kaplan(2) reported that there was evidence of morbid grief if parents enshrine the effects of the deceased. According to that criterion, about half our families fit this category. In our study, two in the two-year group kept the room the same and kept all of the child's belongings. One infant's room was as it had been, the crib in place, the toys still there, and everything exactly the same. The room of an eighteen-year-old boy who had died still had his schoolbooks on the desk. Everything seemed to be as it had been, almost as though he were coming home.

We also looked at symptoms, including feelings of panic,

anger, or guilt, according to the length of time the child was in treatment. The longer the child was in treatment, usually more than two years, the more difficulty the family was having. This is not surprising, since the mother and the child usually leave the father and siblings at home while they come for treatment and stay as long as six or seven weeks at a time of great stress. When the child dies it is more difficult to once again function as a family unit.

We also received information from the parents about the adjustment of the siblings, even though we did not interview them. Forty-five siblings in the six-month group and twenty-seven in the two-year group were included. Parents described their relationship with their other children since the child's death. None of the parents of the six-month group felt that the relationship had worsened and six said it was better; four in the two-year group said it was better. Sixteen families in the six-month group reported having problems with the siblings since the child died, and six in the two-year group reported problems. These problems included depressive withdrawal, school difficulties, and the child not wanting to see a doctor. This number is less than is reported in the literature.

When I asked families about how the remaining children were coping, many of the parents did not know. For example, in answer to a specific question such as, "Does the child have nightmares?" they said they did not think so, but they really were not sure. It was not that they did not have problems but that parents were so absorbed in their own adjustment that they did not know how the children were doing. Sarnoff(5) points out that the mother has all she can do to keep herself going, much less think about emotionally supporting her husband and children. So maybe the reason that these siblings were not reported to have as many problems as is reported in the literature is that the parents were, themselves, having problems and were not noticing the problems of their surviving children.

The parents saw themselves as adjusting very well. Fourteen of the six-month families and eight of the two-year families saw their coping as average or above average. Only three of the six-month families and one of the two-year families reported the use of alcohol or drugs to cope; this is also lower than has been reported.

When we learned that out of the ninety-five families who were eligible only twenty-five would participate in the study, we were surprised that so few were willing to talk with us. We sent a follow-up letter in which we said we respected their right not to participate but would they tell us why they were reluctant. Of the fifty-three letters that we sent out, we received responses from twenty-two people. Half of those families said it was just too tough to talk about their child. This is similar to the earlier finding that, even after two years, there continues to be an emotional response that people do not generally acknowledge. Some families could not manage any contact with us.

How are the St. Jude families doing? We can say that they are grieving longer than we expected, that they are not likely to talk about their child in the early months after the death, that they are likely to have many somatic complaints, and that the preoccupation of mothers with thoughts of their lost child leads to the exclusion of thoughts of others, even the husband and the remaining children. We can say that the longer a family is in treatment with the ill child, the greater the chance of marital problems and that siblings are reported to be better adjusted than other studies have indicated.

What did these families think of the treatment? One hundred percent said that if they had to do it again they would in spite of the fact that they lost their child. Most families saw the years, even though treatment was painful for some, as bonus years that they had with their child that they would not otherwise have had. Most said that what kept them going was the hope that maybe, while their child was receiving treatment, a cure would be discovered.

The limitations of the study are obvious: We had only a twenty-six percent participation rate in spite of the follow-up letters. This was a retrospective exploratory study. Furthermore, we had no knowledge of individual personality structure, previous problems, or coping styles. Our study suggests a need, however, for further exploration of ways that families can be assisted in their grieving so that family integrity can be maintained and unnecessary suffering avoided.

REFERENCES

1. Binger, C. M., Ablin, A. R., Feuerstein, R. C., Kushner, J. H., Zoger, S., & Mikkelsen, C. Childhood leukemia: Emotional impact on patient and family. *New England Journal of Medicine,* 1969, *280,* 414–418.
2. Kaplan, D. M., Grobstein, R., & Smith, A. Predicting the impact of severe illness in families. *Health and Social Work,* 1976, *1,* 71–82.
3. Lascari, A. D., & Stehbens, J. A. The reactions of families to childhood leukemia: An evaluation of a program of emotional management. *Clinical Pediatrics,* 1973, *12,* 210–214.
4. Parkes, C. M. *Bereavement: Studies of grief in adult life.* New York: International University Press, 1972.
5. Sarnoff, Harriet. *The bereaved parent.* New York: Crown, 1977.

unit **B**

FAMILIES AND STAFF:
ERCEPTIONS AND POLICIES

6

parents' perceptions of nursing care of their chronically ill child

AUDREY M. RATH

Audrey M. Rath, RN, MS, now a nurse practitioner consultant for the Arizona State Board of Nursing in Phoenix, believes that listening to parents' perceptions can give insights to staff that lead to improved care. These interviews, conducted and analyzed while Ms. Rath was a research associate in the Department of Pediatrics at the University of Arizona Health Sciences Center in Tucson, give firsthand documentation of the experiences reported by parents in health care settings.

When I asked the parents of chronically ill children to define and describe their perceptions of the nursing care of their children, I wanted to obtain information about the kinds of nursing care parents think are needed but are not being provided(1). At first

I was concerned whether parents would talk to me honestly about the nursing care their child received in the hospital, but I had worked in pediatric nursing a long time and had developed some good relationships with parents. Parents were willing to talk in interviews lasting about an hour. Although I wanted the reactions of both fathers and mothers to nursing care, most fathers turned the interview over to their wives. One said, for example, "You talk to her. I don't want to talk." The interviews were conducted, therefore, with ten mothers from low-income to high-income groups. Their children had a chronic illness, either a cardiac, respiratory, orthopedic, neurologic, or oncologic condition. There were three Mexican-American, one Black, one Native American, one French-American, and four Anglo mothers, all of whom spoke English.

Six of the children had experienced five or more hospitalizations, others from two to four. The mean age of the children was ten years and nine months, ranging from seven years through twelve years and ten months. The mean duration of illness was seven years and eight months, which means the children had been ill over half their life span.

I collected the information through tape-recorded interviews. Three of those interviews were held in a private office; all the rest were held at the bedside because parents wanted to be near their child who would otherwise have been alone in the room. The questionnaire was adapted from an earlier study(2) of perimortality care of oncology patients and their families.

- While your child has been in the hospital he has been receiving nursing care. As far as you are concerned, what is nursing care?
- What kinds of nursing care have been most helpful to your child?
- What kinds of nursing care have been least helpful to your child?
- What other kinds of nursing care would you have wanted for your child?

Most of the mothers said that everything was provided that could possibly be provided for their child. But they suggested that showers in the children's rooms should have bath mats so that children would not slip and fall. They also wanted bars on windows that can be opened from the inside, since on this pediatric unit some of the windows in the rooms could be opened, a fire department rule. One parent was particularly concerned that her child could throw toys out the window or that some child could crawl out the window and fall three stories. Other suggestions were:

- Arrange for roommates approximately of the same age.
- Give some rules to parents when they enter the hospital about proper language used in the hospital and proper use of television.
- Interview older children regarding their likes, dislikes and concerns, when a nursing history is taken.
- Provide books and games for older children in the playroom, which seems to be geared to younger children.
- Establish a list of nursing staff who are proficient in starting intravenous. (Chronically ill children have had many IV's in their lives. Their veins become scarred and collapse easily. If the parents know that the person starting the IV has had some experience or is the most experienced person on the unit, the fears and anxieties of the parents and the child may be allayed.)

The mothers made the following comments about what they considered nursing care to be:

- Making sure that she has the medicine at the time the doctor says, putting the fluids into her, making sure her output is OK.
- It's someone looking after you, his health needs, whatever it happens to be at the time. His health is important, it's whatever needs to be done by someone that knows what they're doing.
- The administration of medicine and care and attention my child receives from the nursing staff.
- Where she has to have special attention and special care for the problem she has. They have to know what they are doing.

- Taking care of their patients, getting involved and doing their job.
- The best medical care my child can get. I expect tops from the nurses. They are very honest, answer questions, are relaxed.
- The nurses coming to help my child mainly with his vital statistics (signs), also helping me take him to the bathroom because he is not able to go.
- Meeting the physical needs of the child . . . but also a child's emotional needs and especially, when it's a child, I think it involves more needs of the family as well.

After each interview was transcribed I underlined what I thought were important points. Then, as certain points began to stand out in each interview, I grouped and labeled them. I then formulated a definition for each group. Six categories emerged: right to know, environment, nutrition, attitude/approach, parent concerns, and competency.

Right to know means the open and honest communication between all members of the nursing team, parents, and child with regard to (a) the status and/or condition of the child, (b) explanations of tasks and/or procedures being performed, and (c) patient education about the disease process, medication, and procedures that may be needed at home. These are some of the statements that the parents made that were used to develop this category:

- I do like to know when my child is taking drugs, and I think I have the right to know the side effects, because I think that's important.
- They didn't tell me that with milk tetracycline is no good. (This child was taking tetracycline at home and nobody had instructed her that tetracycline should not be given at mealtime and with milk, but rather an hour before meals or two hours after meals.)
- They explain to me, and of course they go over it with my child, any procedure that is done. The doctor tells me anything, but when I need to find out some detail or specifics I ask the nurses. Like this afternoon I needed to know what time she was going to physical therapy.

• Here the nurses talk to her, tell her that it may sting or hurt a little bit. That's one thing I like about it, because they explain and try to be as gentle as they can.

Environment is the milieu encompassing the hospitalized child, including the emotional atmosphere, the physical surroundings, and the human resources. Some of the statements regarding these properties were:

• This is a more relaxed place, you don't have the impression you're in jail.
• I feel pretty relaxed, I can talk to the nurses pretty freely, and I can go into some of the other patients' rooms and talk to the parents.
• They take her to the cafeteria and things like that. They take her downstairs to the gift shop.
• He can go outside. At most hospitals when they are doing tests they don't let you outside, and he can walk around the hospital, which is really great.
• We can come anytime and his aunts and uncles have been able to come without being told, 'You have to leave. No more than two persons in the room.' Her sister comes in and visits her. She can do pretty much what she would do at home.

In addition to wanting people close to their child, parents also noted the importance of a playroom and play therapy for their children:

• Here it's very colorful, you have a nice colorful playroom.
• She never wanted to go to the playroom, I guess she didn't feel like playing, but after she started getting better that's all she wanted to do.

Nutrition includes those aspects of care involving food and fluids served to the hospitalized child. Nutrition encompasses food preparation, palatability, food preference, and serving size. Although other categories had a balance of positive and negative comments, this category had more frequent negative comments than positive ones. These negative comments may have been due to the decreased appetite that an ill child experiences, to the change from the food usually eaten at home, and also to the fact that sometimes the medicine can have side effects such as nausea and vomiting. Some of the comments were:

- My food is a lot spicier. . . . No taste, she wouldn't eat it because she's used to having her food served with seasoning and also salt.
- Very tasteless, very. The hamburgers are tasteless. The wax beans are greasy.
- My child said, 'I don't like the food, it tastes lousy. It sits out there for a half-hour before they serve it to me and it is cold.'
- They have the same food every morning for breakfast. There's only certain kinds of cold cereal that she'll eat, and they don't have those here.
- There are no beans or tortillas.
- He got a small breakfast the other morning.

Attitude/approach pertains to the characteristics of the staff behavior toward the parents or child; this includes compassion, friendliness, and trust. Some of the comments were:

- You can pick out nurses who you feel really want to sit down and listen, and they are really concerned for that child, are compassionate.
- You wish the nurse who really feels and cares about your child is going to kind of mother him when you are not there. You know, can I just kind of be your mother for today or tonight, or whatever, so the child can feel that they can tell the nurse what is bothering them, or something that is worrying them, instead of the mother.
- The nurses are rushed. Sometimes it seems it's "Hi" and "Bye" and "I don't have the time." I think the morning ones are too busy. It's hectic in the morning here. Everybody running around.

- I feel very comfortable leaving at night. I know she's all right and I know I would be notified at any time and I can call in during the night at any time.

Parent concerns pertain to those aspects of care with which the parents have an uneasy state, apprehension, or uncertainty regarding the care of their child. Parent concerns are such issues as individualized care, staffing, and enough time to rest. Some of the comments were:

- I wonder whether anyone, whether the nurses, kind of talks with the child to find out what they like and what they don't like, what bothers them the most.
- Do the nurses talk with them and learn things about them like how many brothers and sisters they have, and what he likes to do at school, or this kind of thing?
- Now this child has been sick and he is tired and needs his rest and yet all of the treatments are delayed.
- I'm feeling that my child's biggest complaint is that he is not getting enough rest. The treatments run rather late at night and begin early in the morning and with the other disturbances that come in between, he is not resting well.

Competency, the last category, is actually composed of two subcategories.

One is staff competency, pertaining to how parents perceive the expertise of the nursing staff performing any task, duty, or procedure. This subcategory includes skills, personnel availability, and responsiveness to needs. Statements about staff competency were:

- Well, as far as her medication, my gosh, they're always very punctual. With her bath and everything.
- My child doesn't need any more medication for pain now, but when she did it was very hard to get hold of the nurse.
- I rang the bell and they came right away and they changed her, even in the middle of the night.

The other subcategory is parent competency and pertains to those aspects of care that are provided by the parents and their expertise regarding the child's care and condition, including the credibility of their reports and comments. Comments parents made regarding their own care of their child were:

- I give her the medicine and I bathe her and I get her up when she needs to be got up.
- They taught me quite a bit, and if it weren't for them teaching me so I could do it at home, my child wouldn't be as strong as she is now.
- Maybe it's that they feel that after they bring them out of ICU, they should be well enough to be up on their own, on their own feet. But there's just something I don't like about it. (This mother gave a lot of nursing care to her child after the child came out of ICU because she thought the nurses weren't paying enough attention to her child.)
- I gave them a hard time, very hard time sometimes. His veins are not good and it's better if they take and support his under-arm. His veins are rubbery, sometimes it works better if you put your hand under here, and sometimes when they can't get the blood to flow, if they take the tourniquet off, then the blood flow will come faster. (This mother had a lot of experience with having IVs started on her child, and she was quite expert on what worked and what did not work.)

It is clear that the parents can help the nursing team. They have definite standards that they formulate and compare nurses against from one hospitalization to another. The nurses' attitude and approach, as well as their competency, is very important. A colorful, cheerful atmosphere is also important to the family and to the child.

After the interviews were completed I compared my results with other studies(3, 4), particularly one by Hampe(3), that identified eight needs of grieving spouses in the hospital setting. When I looked at my categories they were similar to the eight categories she indicated, except for number five, the need to be informed of the impending death. Since none of the children in my interviews were near death, that was one need I did not expect these parents to have. Everything else was identified: the need to be with the patient and the need for the comfort and support of family members (environment); the need to be helpful to the patient and the need for assurance of the comfort of the patient (competency); the need to be informed of the condition of their child, the patient, (right to know); the need for acceptance, support, and comfort from health professionals (attitude/approach); and the need to ventilate emotions. After several of the ten interviews that I conducted, the mothers continued to talk with me after the tape recorder was shut off for an hour or more about their family, transportation, insurance, finances, and other kinds of problems that they needed to discuss. Since I was available, the parents felt free to satisfy their need to talk.

I would recommend that interviews such as these be conducted regularly and that fathers be interviewed as well. This would permit both parents to unburden themselves and share their concerns. The hospital staff members could then learn how their care is perceived.

REFERENCES

1. Rath, A. M. *Parents' perceptions of nursing care of their chronically ill children.* Unpublished Master's thesis. Tucson: University of Arizona, 1979.
2. Atwood, J. *A grounded theory approach to the study of perimortality care and other considerations.* Unpublished Report to the Nursing Department, University Hospital, Arizona Health Sciences Center, Tucson, 1975.
3. Hampe, S. O. Needs of the grieving spouse in a hospital setting. *Nursing Research,* March–April 1975, 24, 11+.
4. Molter, N. C. Needs of relatives of critically ill patients: A descriptive study. *Heart and Lung,* 1979, *8,* 332–339.

7

parental responses to a painful procedure performed on their child

MARILYN SAVEDRA

Marilyn Savedra, DNS, Assistant Professor at the University of California, San Francisco, describes the results and implications of her study of parents' behavior and coping strategies to assist their children during blood drawings. Issues concerned with having parents present during painful clinic procedures are considered here.

Should parents be present when their children undergo painful procedures? Does parental presence facilitate or disrupt the accomplishment of the procedure? Do parents want to be with their children when something painful is done? These questions frequently pose a dilemma for those involved in health care delivery to children. Some encourage parents to be with their children; they emphasize the importance of having parents present during medical procedures(1, 2, 3) and urge that the stress of the procedure not be compounded by the stress of separation from the parents. Only "when the parents are unable to provide emotional support for the child" and "when the child is undergoing major surgery" should parents be refused the opportunity to be with their child(4). When procedures are difficult to perform, parental presence is also considered disruptive and may cause delay in accomplishing what must be done, adversely affecting the children, the parents, and the health professionals(5). Other professionals believe children have increased stress when parents "allow" pain or assist in inflicting pain, even though they recognize the value of parents staying with their children.

Seldom are parents asked what they feel is best for their child.

BACKGROUND

There is a paucity of research to guide health professionals in making decisions about parental presence when a child must have a painful procedure. In one study(6) of the effects of separation from their mothers on 112 preschool children in the dental office, children whose mothers remained with them had a more positive response. The mother's presence did not have a deleterious effect on the child's behavior. No studies were found that asked parents if they wanted to remain with their child during a painful procedure.

Pain is unwanted and stressful regardless of its intensity or duration. Anna Freud(7) described the child in pain as feeling "maltreated, harmed, punished, persecuted, threatened by annihilation." These feelings are heightened in the young child when the pain results from an intrusive procedure. With an inability to conceptualize what is inside the body, the child believes the skin is holding the body together, so any penetration of the skin, in addition to being painful, is viewed as dangerous.

THE PROBLEM DEFINED

Because there is little information about parents' behavior and feelings when they are with their child during a painful procedure, an exploratory study was designed to describe parents' behavior when their child's blood was drawn. Blood withdrawal is a procedure commonly performed on children and is assumed to be painful. Most parents have experienced blood drawing themselves so the procedure is not unfamiliar. The study sought to answer the following questions:

- What strategies do parents use to help their children cope with the situation?
- What factors influence how the parent responds?
- Do parents wish to be present when their children are having blood drawn?
- What do parents find difficult about the experience?
- What would parents like health professionals to do for them when parents are with their children during blood withdrawal?

METHODOLOGY

Parents of sixty children two weeks to six years of age who were having blood drawn in a pediatric clinic consented to participate in the study. Parents of children with a major chronic illness necessitating regular intrusive procedures and children with terminal illness were excluded from the study.

Forty-five of the sixty were observed in a large county hospital, which provided greater access than the other observation setting, a pediatric clinic in a medical center. In both settings, however, parents were expected to stay with their child. Blood was drawn in rooms designated for that purpose. Infants were placed on an examining table or the parents' laps. At the medical center children sat on a stool facing a table, and at the county hospital children sat on a chair with an arm rest. Older children who were resistant were placed on the examining table. Blood was drawn in both settings by a laboratory technician who was regularly assigned to the area. The technicians were skilled in performing the procedure and appeared confident. In both settings the technicians were warm and personable, but they gave a minimal explanation regarding the procedure to the child or parent. They were tolerant of the young child's behavior and gave no indication of personal distress. At the medical center pictures of babies covered the table top, while at the county hospital a mobile hung from the ceiling, a large animal picture was on the wall, and one window faced the courtyard. The county clinic served clientele primarily from a lower socioeconomic class. The medical center clients were from all socioeconomic levels.

Data were collected by participant observation and parent interview. Parents who came with their young child to the pediatric laboratory were told the author was interested in finding out what it was like for parents to be with their child when blood was drawn. Permission was requested to observe the procedure and to ask them a few questions immediately thereafter. Although no parent refused to be observed, some gave varying reasons why they could not stay to answer questions. These parents were not pressed to participate and were not included in the study. The interview was conducted following the procedure, after the parents had comforted the child and had given cues of readiness. Most parents were eager to share their feelings.

Parents were observed before, during, and following the procedure. Parent and child behaviors were recorded immediately after the encounter and before a second observation was begun. The parent interview was conducted following the procedure and before leaving the pediatric clinic. Questions were kept to a minimum since the parents and children were eager to leave the clinic or to complete the clinic visit. The interview questions were pretested on a sample of eight to ascertain the clarity and time involved.

ANALYSIS AND FINDINGS

Tabulation of selected variables revealed that in the majority of observations the mother was the parent who was present $(N = 49)$. Eight children were accompanied by their fathers and both parents were present with three children. Over half the parents had been with their children on previous occasions when blood was drawn $(N = 36)$. The largest number of parents were Caucasian $(N = 26)$, the second largest number Black $(N = 23)$, six parents were Latino, and five were Asian. Slightly more than half of the children were boys $(N = 34)$. Blood was taken from veins $(N = 35)$, fingers $(N = 36)$, and feet $(N = 9)$.

Observational data were analyzed by categorizing behaviors of parents and children. Each observation was divided into three periods: (1) predrawing: time of arrival at the laboratory to the point just before the needle was inserted into the vein or the skin was pricked, (2) during blood drawing: vein or skin prick to the application of a Band-aid or gauze dressing, and (3) postdrawing: immediately following application of a dressing to departure from the blood-drawing area. Four categories of parental behavior were formed and defined as follows:

Verbal

Talking and/or making soothing sounds to the child.

Nonverbal

Physical contact with the child such as rubbing or stroking some part of the body, kissing, holding a hand.

Passive

Standing by or holding the child without overtly making an attempt to touch or talk to the child.

Distress

Overt: States that the event is distressing or makes a comment such as "God" in a distressed tone.

Covert: Nonverbally indicates distress by such behaviors as turning away and grimacing.

Parental strategies for helping the child were broadly differentiated as verbal and nonverbal. Verbal strategies included soothing and/or encouraging remarks, distraction such as "Look at the picture," "Look away," offers of a reward or treat, urging control, or stating the procedure would not hurt. Nonverbal strategies included physical contact such as stroking or holding a hand and offering comfort devices such as a bottle or food.

Behaviors of the children were grouped into four categories using a continuum from no apparent distress to physically resistive:

No apparent distress

Watchful and alert but showing no overt distress as evidenced by verbalizations or physical behavior. (Afterward, may be talkative and active, or quiet with no overt signs of distress.)

Concerned

Does not protest or physically resist, but facial expression is concerned and/or anxious.

Protesting

Cries and/or is verbally resistive, such as "I don't want a shot."

Resistive

Physically tries to withdraw or attack.

Variables noted included the position of the child during the procedure, the presence of another health professional to give support or restraint to a resistive child, and parental knowledge of the reason for the blood being drawn.

Responses to the interview questions were tabulated. Differences between all identified variables were computed using chi square. The behavior of the parents was similar before and during blood drawing. Predrawing, the majority of the parents (65%) talked to their child and made soothing sounds, or they combined talking with physically soothing gestures. Twenty-eight parents (47%) during predrawing and twenty-one parents (35%) during blood withdrawal used nonverbal strategies such as patting, stroking, and holding a hand. Sixteen parents (27%) either held their child on their lap or stood by without talking or physically attempting to soothe their child. Nonverbal strategies increased after blood drawing (20%) as did passive behaviors (43%), while verbal strategies alone decreased (15%).

Although forty-four parents (73%) were noted to talk to their child, we made no attempt to note the quantity of communication. At one end of the continuum was the parent who talked continuously while at the other end was the parent who spoke only a few words. For example, the mother of a boy almost five years of age kept a constant stream of talk, "Keep your arm still; don't move; turn your face; turn your face;" she turned his face with her hands. The child jumped when the stick was made but remained quiet. The mother glanced toward me with a look of relief and resumed her talk, "That's all; you're a brave boy; that wasn't bad."

Fifteen parents (25%) indicated verbally or nonverbally that the experience was distressing. For instance, a mother of a five-year-old who was asked if she would be willing to let me observe and interview her said, "Mother panics. I don't like needles." The child, tearful and clinging, sobbed, "I don't want any shot. I hate to do it." The mother then gave verbal reassurance, squatting to the child's level. She suggested the child choose the finger to be used. Although admittedly she found the needles unpleasant, the mother was responsive to her child. Another mother responded when asked to participate, "It's terrifying. I don't like it." Statistically significant was a difference in race in response to stress $(P < .0012)$. Fewer Caucasian parents than Black, Asian, or Latino indicated distress. Asian parents gave nonverbal more than verbal indications of distress more often than Caucasian parents. Parental distress was also significantly related $(P < .04)$ to the presence of a health professional, such as a pediatric nurse practitioner or a physician. Additional help to restrain resistive children was significantly more often used when parents exhibited distress $(P < .005)$ and when a parent could identify what was hard about being with the child when blood was drawn.

Parents were not overtly disruptive of the procedure. They obediently assisted as directed by the technician or nurse. On three occasions parents were told that it facilitated the procedure when the infant cried and, although it appeared difficult for them to halt their strategies to calm their babies, they did so. Only one mother displayed assertive behavior. As the technician was inspecting the arm, she forcefully asked if the blood had to be drawn from a vein. She said that the baby was too small and active and that it would hurt more. The technician complied and took the blood from the baby's finger. In another instance, a father's request was granted when he asked that the left hand be used since the child was right-handed.

Parental behaviors to emotionally support the child were further categorized into more specific strategies including distraction, comfort devices, offering a reward, urging control of behavior, stating the procedure did not hurt, and providing physical contact. Seventeen parents used distraction, directing the child's attention to the pictures, directing the child to look out of the window, or simply telling the child to turn his face or look away. Six parents urged control by saying, for example, "Don't move." "Sit up for mommy." Two parents offered a treat to follow. One told the child he could say "ouch." Only two parents suggested that there would be no pain.

Most parents' verbal support came in a natural easy flow. A mother of a three-year-old told him to "sit like you are going to eat." He promptly asked if he were going to eat. The mother remarked in a distressed tone, "Oh dear, I shouldn't have said that." More than one-half ($N = 35$) of the parents initiated soothing physical contact. Only one parent was observed to slap the child in an effort to get him to hold still. Eight parents offered some type of comfort device, particularly to small infants and young children, such as a pacifier, bottle, or food. Comfort devices were offered significantly more ($P < .009$) when a vein was used for drawing blood.

No statistically significant differences were found between the strategies of parents and the children's behaviors. During pre-blood drawing, the behavior of twenty-eight (46%) of the sixty children was categorized as positive; they gave no overt indications of distress. Three others (5%) appeared concerned. Nineteen (32%) protested, and ten (17%) were resistive; both behaviors increased during the procedure. Six continued to protest following the procedure, and four were quiet but had an anxious expression on their faces. The remaining fifty (83%) were classified as positive; they became active and talkative or, if quiet, gave no obvious signs of anxiety. One twelve-month-old child sat placidly while his toe was pricked. He watched closely, moving his shoe from hand to hand as the toe was manipulated vigorously to get the required blood. The mother commented that he was a quiet baby and did not cry or react to things like that.

The sex of the parent, race, sex of the child, site of blood withdrawal, and previous parental presence also showed no statistically significant differences. However, the number of fathers compared to mothers and the number of Asian and Latino parents were too small to make any important comparisons. No statistically significant difference was found between the parental behaviors and site of the injection with the exception that comfort devices were used more frequently when the withdrawal site was a vein. However, parents frequently said that use of a vein was more distressing for them.

In retrospect it would have been helpful to have gathered data on what parents usually did to comfort their child when he/she was in pain in other situations. A number of parents did use things in the environment to distract their child before and during the procedure. This strategy might be used more often if objects were more available. No attempt was made to determine past experiences of the parents in relation to blood drawing.

Forty-eight parents, a majority, expressed the desire to be present when their child was having blood drawn. Five additional parents said they wanted to be present for this particular time, but would not under other circumstances, such as when a neck vein was used, or in an emergency situation. Five parents unequivocally said they did not want to be present, and two parents said it made no difference. One mother stated that as her child got older than five years of age, it might be best for him to go in alone. She said she would wait outside and be ready to meet him. She suggested that the experience would be "his thing" and that he would need some privacy. In response to whether they felt it was good to be present, fifty-six parents said yes and four said no. Of the four "no" responses, three had previously said they did not want to be present and one said it made no difference.

The vast majority commented on the benefit of their presence to the child with such statements as: "It helps him." "He's a sensitive child and needs someone he knows." "It gives her comfort." "He'd flip out more without me." "It reassures him." "She'd cry if she didn't see me." Seven parents felt it was good to be present so that they would know what was happening. Parents responded similarly to the two questions, "Do you think there is anything good about being present with your child?" and "Do you feel it helps your child when you are present?" Parents spoke about what they could do. "I can comfort him." "I can hold him against me so he doesn't see and that way he doesn't cry as much." "I can calm him." One parent asserted that she could make sure nothing went wrong, such as a needle breaking, if she were present. The need for the child to have someone to cling to in a threatening situation was expressed. Parents felt their presence was calming in helping the child to feel safe, secure, relaxed, and confident. The importance of the children having someone they know with them was felt by some parents to be helpful.

In response to the question "What is hardest for you when

you are with your child?" twenty parents said nothing was hard. Further elaboration included such comments as "I'm used to it." "He's well." "It wasn't in a difficult place." "It has to be done." and "It doesn't hurt." Of the forty parents who indicated one or more things that were hard for them, fourteen comments were about pain and/or how the child was feeling, eleven were about the child's crying, nine were about "the needle," and three about explaining what was happening to the child.

WHAT PROFESSIONALS CAN DO TO HELP

After much hesitation many parents answered the question, "In your opinion what could nurses and other medical people do to help parents in relation to this experience?" Seventeen, almost a third of the parents, said nothing could be done to help them. Several, with encouragement, did make further comments. The majority of responses could be grouped into two categories. One category related to the skill with which the procedure was done and the other related to the approach taken with the child. Parents wanted the person involved with the blood drawing to "be nice, smile, love, hold the child if he were alone, be patient, comfort the child, reassure the child, be understanding, and be truthful." Six parents wanted to know more about what was being done.

With few exceptions, parents expressed a strong desire to be with their child during blood drawing in an outpatient setting. It was the parents' conviction that the child needed them for emotional support and that their presence was helpful to the child. Many parents expressed the belief that the experience would be more upsetting to the child if denied the presence of a parent.

It cannot be discounted, however, that there were parents who would have preferred, if given a choice, not to be present. Three variables are common to these parents. In all cases the site for blood drawing was a vein. Four of the five parents (in one situation both parents were present) did not feel their presence was helpful to the child, and four had previously been present when blood was drawn. Health professionals need to be more aware of individual differences and intervene accordingly. It may be that these parents need to be made aware of the positive aspects of being present, or they may need to be relieved of this responsibility.

There were parents who were distressed by the experience and either spoke of their discomfort or showed their distress by their facial expressions or body postures. This did not prevent these parents from using strategies similar to the parents who did not overtly indicate their distress. It is impossible, of course, to say how much the parent's feelings influenced the child's response to the experience.

Parents' strategies varied. The vast majority talked to the child. They appeared to sense the threat of the situation to the child and were for the most part tolerant of the child's verbal and nonverbal behavior. Two mothers were being loud and brusque. One told her two-year-old "It's not going to hurt," then commanded "Don't move, Lionel! Don't move!" She watched closely as the blood was drawn. She turned to me, "He usually don't cry." She turned back to watch, "That's a lot, hey!" The child continued to cry louder and tears flowed down his face, "Don't cry. We go see Henry. Be a big boy. She's going to write it all down. You're a crybaby." This was also the one instance when a parent called attention to me during the procedure.

Parents did indicate their expectations as to how their child would behave. The quiet baby, discussed earlier, is a case in point. In another instance a mother of a four-year-old was asked if she would like to hold her child's hand. "No," she replied, "He'll be all right. He's had it done before." Some children, however, were less controlled and less cooperative than on previous occasions. A fifteen-month-old child returned a week after his blood was drawn, at which time the mother had blood drawn. The child began to cry when the needle was inserted into his mother's arm in much the same manner as he had cried when his own blood had been drawn.

The most difficult question for parents to answer in the post-drawing interview was how they felt health professionals could help them. Although a few were articulate, many could give no answer. Either it seemed like a foreign thought to them, or they did not feel comfortable expressing their feelings. The predominant theme of those who did elaborate was that a warm, caring approach helped the child most. A small number expressed a desire for information.

In summary, the data obtained from observing and talking to parents who were present at the time of blood drawing indicated that parents use a variety of strategies to help their children cope. They are not disruptive of the procedure. Even when the experience is difficult and stressful, they support their children and assist as directed by the medical personnel. Most parents wish to be present. There is some indication, as evidenced by the children's behaviors following blood drawing, that the parent's presence is helpful.

Further research is needed regarding parental presence during other painful procedures such as spinal taps and changing burn dressings, during procedures performed in different settings, and during procedures when the child is acutely or chronically ill. More information is needed about the indicators that influence personnel to deny parental presence at certain times when they are usually supportive of parental participation. When these data are available more appropriate decisions can be made regarding parents' involvement during painful procedures performed on their children.

REFERENCES

1. Fagin, C. M. Why not involve parents when children are hospitalized? *American Journal of Nursing,* June 1962, *62,* 78–79.
2. Bellack, J. Helping a child cope with the stress of injury. *American Journal of Nursing,* August 1974, *74,* 1491–1494.
3. Klinzing, D. R., & Klinzing, D. G. *The hospitalized child: Communication techniques for health personnel.* Englewood Cliffs, NJ: Prentice-Hall, 1977.
4. Ibid. page 76.
5. Waechter, E. H., & Blake, F. G. *Nursing care of children.* Philadelphia: J. B. Lippincott, 1976, pp. 121–122.

6. Frankl, S. N., Shiere, F. R., & Fogels, H. R. Should the parents remain with the child in the dental operatory? *Journal of Dentistry for Children,* 2nd Quarter, 1962, 150–163.
7. Freud, Anna. The role of bodily illness in the mental life of children. *Psychoanalytic Study of the Child,* 1952, 7, 76.

8

rituals of the
hospital culture

MAXENE JOHNSTON

Maxene Johnston, RN, MA, is Director of Ambulatory Services at Childrens Hospital of Los Angeles. As a pediatric nurse anthropologist she suggests rethinking the communication styles and roles found in most hospitals in order to acknowledge their impact on the patient and family and to design more effective and appropriate communication.

A hospital exists as a complex of elaborate subcultures, a microcosm of aspects of our larger society, a constantly shifting social order with conflicting value systems and widening gaps in communication(1). Physicians, nurses, administrators, and patients comprise separate categories or subcultures; each group has its own values, language, role perceptions, and goals. With the addition of subcultures of technicians and other professionals necessary to the operation of the hospital, there is the beginning of a complicated and confusing social organization.

STAFF AND PATIENT SUBCULTURES

We now know that cultural practices introduced from alien cultures are either accepted, modified, or rejected to the degree that they are compatible with the forms and meanings of the host culture. For our purposes the host culture is the hospital. With the diverse cultures found in a hospital community, staff and patients often have difficulty relating to and accepting each other since they have different purposes and goals. Furthermore some of the values and goals of one particular group conflict and are incompatible with those of the other. For example, although cleanliness is an important value to the staff, patient waiting time usually is not.

The various professional participants in the hospital culture may not be aware of conflicts since the language through which values and goals are communicated has different meanings for each group. Evaluating a patient at home, for example, is referred to as a *house call* when performed by a physician and a *home visit* when carried out by a nurse. Patients may be reluctant to bring children they believe to be sick to scheduled appointments in a "well-baby" clinic. Parents will also resist discussing their children's behavioral problems if the practitioner is oriented to physical growth and apparently uninterested in psychosocial care. In these ways a hospital can be like a foreign country, with alien customs, language and schedules to which patients and families must adapt(2).

PREPARING THE HOSPITAL TO ADAPT TO THE PATIENT

Even though much has been said and written about the importance of preparing the patient in order to reduce the negative effects of hospitalization, such preparation is often neglected, especially for those who have had prior hospitalizations. Perhaps this is because it is assumed that a patient who has already been there is familiar with hospital staff, treatments, and rituals and is known by the hospital staff. Yet, observations at a large rehabilitation hospital showed that it was not unusual to see a young child clinging to his mother after being readmitted to the hospital. At times a child with a history of multiple hospitalizations for orthopedic surgery, physical therapy, or surgical revisions of former work would become physically uncontrollable when approached by a nurse or doctor. Other children indicated distress by withdrawal, by shutting out a very threatening kind of world. Children still react to an intrusive procedure as if it were an invasion or an attack, even though they have been through it before. They do not react with increased familiarity or adaptation to repeated surgery or transfer to a second hospital, a common occurrence with children who have chronic illnesses. On the contrary, sensitized by their initial experience it is not uncomon for them to experience a high degree of tension and nervousness when confronted with the varied rituals, customs, costumes, and vocabularies of various hospitals.

It is a surprise to many to learn of the meaning children have assigned to hospital routines. Some children have said that blood tests were taken to weaken them so that they could not move, that oxygen masks were used to muffle their screams, and that intravenous fluids were given to sedate them. One eleven-year-old insisted that the cast room was where arms and legs were cut off, and other children have refused to cooperate with the inhalation therapist because they believed that "only dying kids get oxygen."

The admitting process itself is a routine that warrants examination. This frequently involves many phases and several hospital departments. In Karachi, Pakistan, this routine is so ceremonious that Dr. Hasan of the Jinnah Postgraduate Medical Center calls it "the bridal procession of the patient," or "marrying the patient to the institution," as reported in Bell's study of admission customs(3). He reports also that the admission process provides hospital staff with a chance to relate to family members, sometimes the only such opportunity during the whole course of the patient's illness. Some hospitals take advantage of this occasion; others, however, concentrate on the patient and ignore the families.

Observations of children's admissions in many hosptals revealed typical admitting routines that are chaotic in nature and result in isolating families. Children and parents arrive on the ward at the busiest time of the day when treatments and medications are being given, and often the child's bed is not yet available. With this type of environment it is not difficult to see how the child and family can feel like unwelcome visitors. This introduction does not help families share their concerns, unique needs, or problems. Instead, such a beginning creates a distance between the staff and the child and the parents that lasts throughout the entire hospital period.

Another routine encountered in a medical setting is the clinical evaluation, during which a patient "buys" a diagnosis that may eventually necessitate admission. These evaluations often appear to be ritualistic and standardized in terms of expected behavior of both the patient and the practitioners. Patients and practitioners develop forms of action and behavior that are repetitive and can, therefore, be considered ritualistic. These ritual actions appear to protect against internal antisocial drives that cannot be exhibited publicly. It is as if ritual actions can assure social harmony between staff and patient groups in those situations where harmony is most jeopardized. It upsets the equilibrium too much to do otherwise, so we have certain standards, rules of behavior when we go through our preadmission process. This was evident in several hundred visits I observed in various large, urban, medical centers.

The practice of the "physician first" examination was one such preadmission ritual. Children and families often waited long periods of time for the physician to see them before any other member of the health team could see them. This practice tended to reinforce the belief that outpatient visits are disease- or physiologically-oriented and therefore the primary responsibility of the physician. This ritual also helped to maintain the social harmony between various practitioner groups, since the doctor came first, then the occupational therapist, or the social worker, or the physical therapist, or the child life worker.

In order to examine routine patient-care practices and to modify and adapt such individual patient practices, a pilot clinic program was developed in the pediatric outpatient department of

Rancho Los Amigos Hospital in Downey, California. Until that time it was the patient group that was expected to make the adaptations and adjustments to comply with the general hospital culture. We have all heard staff comment, "He's coming to our hospital; he'll learn our rules here."

Developing a pilot clinic program included the use of community volunteers who served in the role of a culture broker. We also changed the traditional physician-focused organizational protocols and the territorial boundaries observed among members of the caregiving staff. Establishing a family preparation clinic enabled the staff to assume some responsibility for adapting hospital routines to individual patients, thereby minimizing the stress of the situation.

Upon arrival in the clinic, families were met by a preparation volunteer or "culture broker" trained to serve in this capacity. She accompanied the patient and parents through a maze of diagnostic departments that were located some distance from the clinic and helped them negotiate their way through long waiting lines, interpreting procedure and the process the child was experiencing. She was seen by families as belonging to the patient culture while at the same time having the knowledge and privileges afforded only to staff groups. She had a uniform and was allowed some access in the hospital that was not available to the patient. Since the volunteer was a community person and did not belong to any particular hospital subculture she did not incur intrinsic intergroup conflicts. On those occasions when the volunteer did experience conflict she usually identified with the patient culture and used her access to staff to lessen areas of conflict by discussing problems directly with them. Here are some examples to illustrate the kind of miscommunication that a "culture broker" volunteer can correct.

When preadmission diagnostic studies on some children were not being obtained and completed before admission the inpatient staff blamed the outpatient staff. "They can't get anything organized in those clinics. They never know where they put those reports." The physician blamed the hospital administration's poorly organized admitting procedure. The outpatient staff blamed the parents, who, they said, did not understand the instructions given to them regarding the tests. "If those parents would only learn to read. . . ."

After the new clinic began, the volunteer observed and reported that the problem of the missing diagnostic studies came about because families were being instructed to use a particular clinic elevator to find their way to the diagnostic units of the hospital. It was impossible for them to get to where they were supposed to go, however, because another department in the hospital had locked the elevators because of problems with thefts in that particular area. No notice had been given to other departments regarding the inaccessibility of the elevators. Since no one from the clinic had ever accompanied the parents, we did not know where we were sending them. We only thought we knew.

The volunteer also observed and identified the difficulties that parents and babies were experiencing with routine laboratory procedures to obtain blood. The parents did not ask us why blood drawings for three tests were done when the child was coming in for one, but the volunteer whom we had sensitized to the issues of traumatic procedures on children questioned this procedure. An investigation revealed that specimens were being obtained by the venapuncture method rather than by what had been presumed, the finger stick method. This discrepancy was brought to the attention of the appropriate department supervisors who were unaware that an inappropriate approach for obtaining a specimen from their patients was being done, and they soon corrected it.

There is always reason to remain cautious when dealing with an individual who can freely move between two cultural groups. The culture broker is in a position to gain information and expertise and to accumulate power. At this time, however, the influence of the culture broker concept has had a positive impact on the delivery of patient care and has not been disruptive. The social harmony between professional groups and patient groups is improving and will continue to do so with increased competence and knowledge.

The traditional physician-focused organization of the patient visit was changed by having a nurse and social worker begin work with the family immediately upon their arrival, thus eliminating long waiting periods for the patient. It was planned that the physician would follow and complete the necessary history and physical examination of the child. However, changing the traditional "physician first" ritual generated resistance from the physicians. It was now the physician group who found themselves waiting, and they did not like that. After all, they had things to do; they had matters of importance to attend to. The resistance abated when an agreement was made that the physicians would be called to the clinic after other staff members were finished and when the patient was ready to be seen by them.

Finally the family preparation clinic brought the inpatient staff into the clinic setting and the clinic staff became directly involved in the admission process onto the wards. On many occasions when families were called to be reminded of their appointment in the family clinic, we learned that they had changed their minds about surgery or had moved from the area.

The new system enables the clinic nurse to identify many children with suspected or confirmed minor infections. Early identification makes it possible to schedule other children who need procedures and to use efficiently the surgical time assigned in the operating room. The new system enables families to save paying an admitting fee for children who would be discharged when their minor illnesses were assessed on the ward.

The postsurgical intensive care unit nurses are now also attending the family preparation clinics to learn about the children while the children learn about the staff. We have seen beautiful things happen as a result of this. The children are not traumatized, because they are not being admitted that day. We note that the children are more at ease when they are admitted about three or four days later. Children sleep better in the intensive care unit. When they wake up they see the face of somebody they have seen before at the clinic when they were not scared and at a time when they were not about to be separated from their mothers or fathers, they are more trusting.

Staff adapt hospital routines to individual needs in other ways as well. Visiting hours are more flexible. Parental preferences are heard and supported. Children's requests for such things as special pajamas or privacy are being granted. It is hard to believe that these things are still issues, yet we all know that they are.

The more success staff and patient groups have with such programs, the more risks they will likely be willing to take to generate similar adaptations. Moving beyond established functional boundaries within the hospital will facilitate communication and help to resolve problems.

BENEFITS OF CHANGES

During the initial nine months of looking at such changes, several observable benefits were noted. First, families experienced less waiting time in diagnostic departments. What previously had taken up to four hours was now completed in one-and-a-half hours. Second, families were less confused about where to go for various services within the hospital and more willing to obtain preadmission diagnostic studies. Third, more information was exchanged in response to parental concern about separation, care of children after discharge, and the like. Fourth, children were given time and encouragement to express their feelings and received reassurance and information about medical procedures. And last, there was more contact with the day-to-day caregiving members of the staff as well as an opportunity to begin trusting relationships with them, rather than continuing to foster the "unwelcome visitor" role.

Evaluating hospital practices, routines, and rituals and incorporating planned change into the hospital have resulted in several therapeutic benefits for the patient reentering this subculture. Staff groups have become more familiar with the unique needs and values of patient groups, and children and their families have had less of a tendency to deal with the staff as being from an alien culture. The notion of a hospital being similar to a foreign country is one reality that will, however, require ongoing attention.

REFERENCES

1. Singer, P. The hospital Babel. *Nursing Clinics of North America*, 1970, *5*, 279–288.
2. Gellert, E. Reducing the emotional stresses of hospitalization for children. *American Journal of Occupational Therapy*, 1958, *12*, 125–129.
3. Bell, J. E. *The family in the hospital: Lessons from developing countries.* Bethesda: National Institute of Mental Health, 1969.

9

fact or fantasy
about culture

ANN R. SLOAT, CATHERINE DALY,
KATHERINE O'REILLY, DOROTHY CONWAY,
LORRAINE STRINGFELLOW, AND ROY SMITH

*The authors are from the School of Public Health at the University
of Hawaii at Manoa in Honolulu. **Ann R. Sloat, RN, MSN,** served as
convenor and moderator for the panel and begins this paper by
describing themes in the presentations of **Catherine Daly, MSW,
MPH; Katherine O'Reilly, MPH; Dorothy Conway, RD, MPH; Lorraine Stringfellow, RN, BSN, MPH; and Roy Smith, MD, MPH.***

As health care providers for families it is imperative for us to be
aware of and to understand the concept of culture, without
stereotyping the beliefs of families, and then to transfer this concept into practice. The egocentricity of children makes them unaware of differences between their culture and that of the
dominant health system they enter as patients. If we, as providers,

are not aware, we may jeopardize the parents' ability to minister to their children's needs, especially when the family's values and belief system are in conflict with ours and not reflected in care. The papers that follow point to this need for sensitivity to cultural and ethnic differences and similarities.

In the first section, Ms. Daly challenges the reader with the concept that the health provider is a member of a subculture, defined not by ethnicity but by training and socialization into a profession. It is this culture, full of values, rituals, and belief systems, that the health professional needs to be aware of, in order to differentiate and analyze, despite the difficulties of doing so.

Ms. O'Reilly then discusses the responses of parents from different ethnic groups to the experience of having a handicapped infant. The data from this enrichment project emphasize that, although there are differences among ethnic groups, most parents want the best care for their children and have needs in common that cross ethnic and cultural lines.

In the third section Ms. Conway relates the importance, meaning, and uses of family food with various cultures and suggests ways that hospital food can be adapted to accommodate cultural preferences.

Ms. Stringfellow then describes a cultural assessment tool through a case study in which values of a family are contrasted with those of a health provider. It becomes clear in the use of the tool that there are many attitudinal, value-based influences on health behaviors that, when the health professional understands them, become an important constructive element in the care of children and their families.

In the final section Dr. Smith applies the concept of cultural influences on the health practices of families in developing countries as well as to those of the technologically advanced medical world. He suggests that recognizing universal family values about promoting optimum health care can give one a useful perspective in which to view cultural practices.

Since culture is a dynamic concept, rather than a fixed or static state, all of us assimilate and test values and behaviors that were at first foreign to us. Sensitivity to our own values and beliefs as health care providers may be the most important step in appreciating other methods of caring. Such appreciation is necessary for quality health care delivery.

THE CHALLENGE OF THE CONCEPT OF CULTURE

Providing culturally sensitive service is a major issue in health care delivery today, since cultures are a source of values and beliefs that influence consumer health behavior(1, 2).

We see these external traits of the consumer as barriers to care, whereas the real obstruction to care may lie in our own values and attitudes, which are often less susceptible to rational thought and examination. Professional health workers have their own culture values that influence their behavior. The culture of our upbringing and the values of our professional subculture have as much impact on service delivery as the culture of the consumer, perhaps more.

Since hospitalization is a critical experience for families, it is most important that health care professionals be sensitive to their own and the families' cultural variations and values about health, child rearing, and family life.

Although there is generally an attitude of broad acceptance of diverse cultural values, translating stated attitudes about culture into practice presents difficulties. One difficulty is the denial that cultural differences exist at all. Such a belief can lead to misunderstandings, feelings of exasperation, and premature judgments by both health providers and consumers. Romanticizing or overemphasizing cultural differences, on the other hand, can result in feelings of frustration and in the design of faulty systems of care that are based on invalid assumptions about people. Both denying and romanticizing limit the health providers' ability to recognize and support the individuality of families, thereby limiting needs assessment and effective communication.

When we talk about culture we mean that particular constellation of qualities people have acquired and assimilated into their personalities as a result of membership in a given social or ethnic group. Such groups are strong factors that link people in a heterogenous society. However, common educational experiences, similar work patterns, and geographical proximity also cause people to cluster in cultural groups. Thus we can speak of health workers in a hospital as being members of a professional culture, who share similar values and attitudes. Individual personalities and lifestyles may vary, but the institutionally sanctioned norms of efficiency, rationality, organization, styles of dress, and language are shared by people working together in a self-contained, well-defined geographic location.

Both professional and ethnic cultures provide norms that affect decisions about what is right or wrong, appropriate or inappropriate, desirable or undesirable. There are various ways, within different cultural contexts, of expressing the absence of being well, since the recognition of symptoms often reflects culturally learned behavior. In some cultural groups illness may not be viewed as a "temporary setback" to be attacked rigorously in order to effect a cure. Samoan children in Hawaii, for example, who spend a great deal of time at the beach, fishing and swimming, experience chronic skin and ear infections, since the ocean contains coral and volcanic rock with bacteria and other organisms. Samoan parents do not usually seek medical attention at an early stage because these infections are considered normal conditions of childhood. Health personnel, however, are dismayed and discouraged by the parents' apparent lack of responsibility and concern for the children when medical attention is not sought until severe otitis media or impetigo appear.

The concern that both the professional and the family have for the welfare of the child can be obscured by problems stemming from differences in the meaning of words, differences in interpreting health and illness, and differences in cultural remedies. Concepts such as prevention, early intervention, independence and self-reliance are culture bound. Varied understandings and values about these concepts create misunderstandings, causing barriers to communication with patients and limiting access to and use of health care.

When staff stereotype certain ethnic groups and erroneously assess parents as ignorant, lazy, or uncaring, their judgments cause difficulties for the family. The values of health care workers are frequently middle class, characterized by a sense of individual responsibility, competitiveness, and moral certainty. These values are reinforced by professional training and then considered to be based on "expertise." In the accompanying sense of territoriality children can become "our patients" rather than the family's child.

It may be difficult for professionals to recognize parental authority in the care of children. This is particularly true when parents hold a value system or culture that is markedly different from our own. We tend to respond to qualities in parents that are familiar to us and that we can interpret in our own frame of reference. For example, when we remove decision making from parents they may become submissive, which we then stereotype as a particular group's tendency to be dependent and apathetic in the care of their children.

To the professional, health is a top priority. To many people other values have priority in their lives. The chronic "no shows" or the parent who does not cooperate with a prescribed health regimen may be seen as selfishly irresponsible and the behavior perceived as a direct challenge to the health worker's expertise. But many people agree to a medical regimen simply to be polite. Their lack of follow-through is more a lack of agreement on priorities than a lack of concern for their children.

Health professionals in a hospital setting constitute a majority culture. The patient who enters the system is in the minority. If the family cannot adjust "successfully" to the system, they are viewed as irresponsible, as lacking the proper future-orientation, and as holding little value for preventive health care. Compliance or following orders becomes a major issue. When the patient and family who are competent elsewhere are judged out of context, they are assumed to be exhibiting inherent character traits, rather than responding to a stressful situation.

Though staff needs to be aware of varied cultural values, we can become oversensitive to cultural differences. When culture becomes a unique social phenomenon, individuals are perceived as exotic objects rather than as people. This results in a dehumanized system of health care that is not responsive to people's needs.

Heightened awareness of cultural differences between the consumer and professional may tend to isolate the consumer and interfere with communication.

Attributing special needs to people on the basis of the ethnic or social group can deny variations among people who are members of the same group. Similarly, grouping people's needs on the basis of such assumptions can result in a denial of individual expertise and competency. One example then becomes representative of the entire group. Labeling can lead to fallacious conclusions. Some things may be more culture specific, such as food; however, our ability to recognize and utilize this knowledge will be limited if we cannot sort out real from assumed need.

The issue is not whether we design special services for different cultural groups, but on what basis the services are designed. If the design of services is based on professional assumptions about family needs as a function of ethnic or class differences, then we are guilty of stereotyping. The following cliches are all too common: "They can only work with their own kind." "They only respond to a concrete service." "They'll take all they can get." "They're all alike."

The meaning of behavior becomes critical when one accepts that all behavior is purposeful and directed toward attainment of goals. Behavior may then be considered a manifestation of the individual culture. If the behavior is a response to a specific situation, however, the behavior may not reflect parental aspirations or goals.

The responsibility rests with professionals to recognize the meanings and similarities in values regardless of observed behaviors and to understand the role of values in health care.

Professionals expect that parents will adapt to the established norms of the health system, that the parents will modify their values and discard elements of their culture in order to be consistent with our professional value system. The challenge of the concept of culture is to recognize that there are universal parental values of concern and commitment to children. Our professional assessment should be based on understanding the meaning of behavior. Only by seeking meaning to behavior will we be able to relate to the needs, wants, and hopes of families.

Health care should not be colored by an adversary relationship based upon a perception of "them" and "us." Rather, it should be a cooperative relationship based on mutual trust and desire for understanding.

Cultural diversity offers a potential to enrich and enhance work with children and families. Our responsibility as health professionals is to recognize and understand the individual behaviors and needs within cultural groups in order to facilitate the delivery of optimal health care, and to utilize the potential that cultural diversity offers to enrich and enhance work with children and families.

AN ENRICHMENT PROGRAM FOR HANDICAPPED INFANTS

Handicaps do not discriminate. Infants with handicaps come from practically all the ethnic groups in Hawaii. The parents of these infants express similar feelings about their children. There is a universality about caring, but a diversity of ways to express it.

In our enrichment program 110 infants were served within a three-year period. Then the project was disseminated throughout the state. The staff provided training and collected data on 390 children who were served in seven of the state's ten infant programs in one year.

Although Hawaii's population has a multitude of cultures, infants with handicaps are overrepresented from the Hawaiian/part-Hawaiian group (26%) compared with their total population in Hawaii (9%). Underrepresented groups are the Japanese handicapped infants (17% compared to 28% Japanese in the total population), Caucasian (32% handicapped/39% in population), and Chinese (2% handicapped/7% in population) . Three other groups have equivalent populations, Filipinos (13% handicapped/12% in population), other Asians (2%/1.5%), and Blacks (1%/1%).

Possible explanations have been sought for the apparent high rate of handicaps in Hawaiian/part-Hawaiian families. There is an increased rate of premature births to single mothers of Hawaiian/part-Hawaiian ancestry, 5.4% compared with .66% for single Japanese mothers and 1.4% for Caucasian. A lack of early prenatal care for Hawaiian/part-Hawaiian mothers may be a contributing factor; only 63% had their first prenatal visit in the first three months of pregnancy. By contrast, 84% of Japanese women and 72% of Caucasian women sought care in the first trimester. Of births to single Hawaiian/part-Hawaiian mothers, 45% were to women less than nineteen years of age. Comparable figures for Japanese women less than nineteen years of age were 34% and for Caucasian women 27%. Thus there are three criteria that place the Hawaiian/part-Hawaiian baby at high risk for handicapping conditions: prematurity; single, young mothers; and lack of early prenatal care(3).

The data collection system we used included measures of both child and parent progress. A questionnaire entitled *The Child Growth and Development Inventory*(4), developed in an attempt to assess changes in parents as a result of program intervention, measures parents' attitudes, skills, and knowledge about child growth and development.

Attitudes about child growth and development were determined by such questions as: how to answer the questions of friends and siblings about the handicapped baby; feelings about parental guilt; and socialization between handicapped and non-handicapped children. Knowledge was measured through questions about sequential development, selection of appropriate toys, and concepts about teaching young children. Skill items related to having parents choose how they would act in a certain situation involving their infant, for example how to teach language, change behaviors, or handle sibling rivalry.

Three ethnic subgroups had sufficient numbers to allow for a comparison of results: Japanese, Caucasian, and Hawaiian/part-Hawaiian. Attitude change (.41) from pre-test (mean of 8.2) to post-test (mean of 8.6) was significant at the .01 level only for the Caucasian population. Japanese and Caucasian subjects showed no significant change in skills but the Hawaiian/part-Hawaiian group demonstrated significant improvement in skills (1.68, significant at the .05 level) . Caucasian mothers had no change in knowledge. The Japanese mothers showed improved knowledge

(2.7, significant at the .05 level) and the Hawaiian/part-Hawaiian showed an improvement in knowledge (3.3, significant at the .05 level). It should be noted that as the Caucasian mothers scored fairly high on the pre-test, they had little opportunity to improve on the post-test. The parent data suggests that involvement in infant programs has resulted in an attitude change in Caucasian parents. The Hawaiian/part-Hawaiian group gained in skills. Japanese and Hawaiian cultural groups improved in knowledge of child growth and development. Therefore, early intervention programs of the type we offered do appear to help parents, but the areas where gains are made seem to differ according to cultural background.

All families, regardless of ethnicity, are interested in promoting achievement and optimal development of their child. It is also universal that families are distressed, overwhelmed, ashamed, guilty, angry, and shocked about the birth of a child with a handicap. Nevertheless, early intervention does make a difference to families; this difference was demonstrated by the improvement shown on a written test and by what they said about the beneficial effects of the program.

Not enough has been done to study the reactions and needs of different cultural groups who have infants with handicapping conditions. The word *handicapped* is not even part of the language in a number of cultures, including Samoan and many Micronesian groups. However, there are universal needs and reactions of all families. Perhaps it is only the method of responding to these needs that varies according to cultural background.

FAMILY FOOD AND CULTURE

Every culture has determined the ways in which foods are to be used. To reject, by facial expression or words, food that is offered is to reject the person and the culture. However, when a food is offered that is not allowed by a person's culture, then the person offering the food is considered to be offensive and the act is considered to be demeaning.

Eating is regarded not only as a way of appeasing hunger or

obtaining nourishment but also as a duty or virtue, as a gustatory pleasure, or as an element in social or religious communion. Food has meanings that are personal, deep-seated and influenced by culture. The food that may signify security may be milk in one culture and rice in another. Love is shown through the giving of culturally determined foods like mom's apple pie or sushi. Healing foods may be represented by chicken soup or pounded breadfruit. Foods also have purely social uses, such as gifts to promote friendship, to show sympathy, or to demonstrate equality, creativity, or status. There is a saying, "Tell me what you eat and I'll tell you who you are."

Cultural food practices come not only from our ethnic, social, and religious backgrounds but also from our peer groups. The type of food served at a five-year-old's birthday party will not be served at the sixteenth birthday party. The cake may be there, but the belongingness foods and status foods will change with age.

Each ethnic group carefully passes on its food ways through the training of children so that each child knows what is considered food and what is not. Children are also taught socially acceptable behavior in relation to food. Thus they come to know what the limits for food refusals are so that the original impulses toward the satisfaction of hunger are transformed into socially acceptable appetites. The likes and dislikes of parents are an important influence on the eating habits of their children.

One cannot assume, however, that because children are from a particular ethnic group they always eat the foods of that culture. In a one-day dietary record of Honolulu high school athletes, only one food was considered a cultural food, rice. A male Filipino tennis player had a dry cereal breakfast and a school lunch, then for dinner ate some leftovers from his mother's cocktail party. A female swimmer of Chinese origin had an American breakfast, a school lunch, and a taco dinner that she bought in a fast-food place. It was difficult to find any food on the diet of a female tennis player of Japanese origin that could be attributed to the Japanese culture. These students were eating the foods of their present status—on the run. A Filipino nursing student reported that she could not remember eating Filipino food as a child. Her mother cooked Filipino food for herself and her husband and American foods—soups, hot dogs, dry cereals, hamburgers—for the children.

We adopt the culture of who and what we are at the present time. Thus we have baby food, foods for preschoolers, foods for Little Leaguer's, teenage foods, and so on, and these practices are true in the various ethnic groups. Some members of all ethnic and racial groups in Hawaii eat fast-food hamburgers.

Although eating patterns are learned, parents and culture are not the only influence(5). Children are conditioned early by the message of television commercials since they spend time with this "baby sitter." The demand of children in the supermarket for certain cereals shows the carryover of this learning. Immigrants buy advertised foods and feel they are Americanizing their children. A young immigrant father proudly told a nutritionist that every day his son had either a fast-food hamburger or fast-food fried chicken and cupcakes.

Early exposure to the school system is another influence on food habits(6). Because of pressure from their children, immigrant mothers from Southeast Asia regularly request recipes from the schools for spaghetti, tacos, and pizza. You can almost tell how long a Caucasian child has been in Hawaii by his increasing rice consumption.

Nutrition education must take into consideration the foods familiar to the child. A day care center that is very proud of its food service invited me to eat with them. The staff are young, vibrant, and interested in health foods. The menu consisted of whole wheat tortillas filled with garbanzos, cheese, and sprouts; raw cauliflower and raw broccoli with yogurt dip; a dessert of orange slices; and milk. It was a nutritious menu. It tasted very good to me, but the children would not eat it. They were mainly from a low socioeconomic group and a culture different from that of the staff. The milk was drunk and the oranges were eaten but the rest of the food was thrown away. Staff remarks such as "Eat your burrito; it's better for you than that awful white bread you eat at home" were ineffective. Children will eat new foods eventually, but they need to have a learning experience along with them. New foods must be introduced in small quantities, and the foods of their home must be treated with respect.

Health foods are in; junk foods are out. The definition of each differs with each culture and age group. In a survey I did of ten-year-olds, children defined their favorite foods, such as hamburgers, french fries, shakes, candy bars, and popcorn, as "good" foods. Their mothers and the professionals defined them as "junk." A few of the children labeled vegetables as junk food. Mothers and professionals tend to label snack foods of cultures other than their own as junk. Health foods varied depending on the culture of the person rating the foods.

In the hospital, nutrition needs may be affected by tension, trauma, and the disease process. Appetite or willingness to eat may be nil because of the setting, medications, and the emotional trauma of the hospitalization.

One way to ensure children will be getting the nutrients they need is to ask parents and children in intake interviews not only the likes and dislikes of the children, but also what foods the children will take under adverse conditions. These foods, such as ice cream bars, shakes, juices and drinks, can then be fortified with missing nutrients. In the hospital, it is easier to change the food than the family. Another way to encourage nutrition is to take advantage of fleeting appetites. As children are able to take in more food, it should be given slowly and deliberately. Too often trays put in front of children have portion sizes that go beyond their appetite, have foods running together, or have mountains of vegetables. With this in front of them children can lose faith in the food system. It is also useful to have family members with the child at meals. After all, mealtime may have been a time of social contact with the family, the only time children were with the whole family. With strangers, they are not hungry, and when alone, they will not eat. Parents know it is easier to encourage a child to select foods from a cafeteria than it is to explain a menu. Why not bring the cafeteria to the hospitalized child? A food wagon with culturally acceptable favorite foods could be available at mealtime for children to make selections. Favorite foods could be frozen in small batches for reheating every day.

Many hospitals in developing countries have family members sleep near the children and prepare their food. Cooking classes are held on the hospital grounds so that mothers can learn about and meet their children's nutritional needs with the food in the home. Since parents often spend long hours in the hospital by their children's side, nutrition education programs for the parents should be undertaken to assure the continued recovery of the children when they return home.

CULTURAL ASSESSMENT

Cultural behavior is based on the values and beliefs of a particular group of people, a way of doing something that is acceptable and effective. This behavior usually is thought to protect the physical, social, and emotional health of the people in the group.

When people from different cultural groups interact, their differing values and beliefs can cause confusion and misunderstanding and result in undesirable behaviors. Producing desirable behavior requires that each group understand the values and beliefs of each other.

The process of identifying specific behaviors and comparing differences is called cultural assessment. From such an assessment an overall plan of care can be developed.

Though many health workers are sensitive to cultural assessment Aamodt(7) suggests that it be part of our overall family assessment. An example given is about a teenage mother who thinks that diaper bags are pretty, but the nurse thinks it is wasteful to spend money on diaper bags. In addition, the mother thinks that bottle-feeding is best for her, but the nurse thinks that breast-feeding will be easier, cheaper, and better for the baby. By pointing out the differences in the values and belief systems of the mother and the nurse, Aamodt showed how the nurse could better understand the mother's behavior. The process of assessing culture is, therefore, of a practical value.

With the following tool, health workers can describe a specific behavior as perceived by a member of the group being served. The tool also requires workers to describe their own behaviors to identify any differences. The health workers are then asked to suggest an approach that will affect their own behavior in future relationships with that group or a member of that group.

First, categories of interest to maternal and child health

workers are listed, including such entries as reproduction, pregnancy, what children mean to the parents, the role of father and mother, and acceptable ways to receive help.

Second, the consumer's responses to these categories are listed. To obtain these, someone might interview or observe a person or family or do a literature review about a group.

Then the health worker responds to the categories.

Similarities and differences can now be identified. Some of the differences in one case we studied were:

- Pregnancy is viewed as a negative incident by the parent but as a planned positive experience by the staff.
- Children are burdens versus life-enriching.
- Help is best received from family and friends versus professionals and agencies.

For each item an approach is then listed. For example:

- Involve in discussions with other teens regarding pregnancy, contraception, parenting skills and roles.
- Include family in planning for hospitalization, care in home, follow-up.

Health care personnel need to support the family's efforts to do what needs to be done in a way that is acceptable to families. By recognizing and submerging their own cultural biases, providers can help families plan strategies to achieve desired health goals. This process will reduce stereotyping and labeling of people or groups, and that support would help achieve the desired outcome, a plan of care.

The cultural assessment tool is a dynamic instrument. It need not be completed all at once. As new information is obtained, entries are made in appropriate spaces and approaches are added or modified as needed. The categories of information can be changed to meet the needs of a particular specialty group, clinic staff, or individual worker such as a nurse, social worker, or occupational therapist. For example, a maternity service might want categories relating to childbearing, whereas the pediatric service might want categories relating to childrearing behaviors.

Following the introduction of this tool at the ACCH conference, the Head Start Program in Hawaii began to use it to look at the ethnic groups their children represent. Beginning entries have been made for Vietnamese, Samoan, Filipino, and Hawaiian families. The approaches they listed offer them specific ways to work with those children in developing the individual educational plans each child requires.

Health professionals have long stated their intent to be cognizant of cultural differences and to modify their approaches to increase the acceptance and effectiveness of treatments. The cultural assessment instrument presented here can be used for thoughtful preparation of care plans that will be meaningful to the consumers. The tool offers a method to identify cultural differences and to suggest approaches that will not impose provider values on the consumer.

CULTURAL INFLUENCES ON THE HEALTH PRACTICES OF FAMILIES

The value of children as a cultural trait has been carefully studied(8) and lends strength to the thesis that there are universal parental concerns for children. Apparent cultural differences are merely the local interpretations and expressions of these values. Parents the world over want the best for their children and want to establish the optimum environment for their children's development. The overt expression of these concerns is determined by the mores of the locale and may seem bizarre or even cruel to others.

Much has been written about religious beliefs that interfere with effective medical care. Most health professionals are familiar with those sects that believe only in so-called natural healing processes and that do not allow scientific intervention. Less attention has been directed toward the culture-related beliefs that are not found in religion but rather in a social context. Even there, culture-related beliefs are understandable and seem appropriate, even when they are based on ignorance, superstition, or misguided concern.

The developing nations, however, do not have a monopoly on such beliefs. Industrialized nations have their share of such practices as well. In some parts of the world the culturally-based barriers to medical practice assume a very great significance. Recently I had the opportunity to observe the effects of cultural tradition and belief on the development of programs intended to enhance the quality and expand the availability of medical care in a tradition-bound society. That society's medical establishment considered the prevalence of nonconstructive primitive customs to be responsible for a major part of the infant mortality and early childhood mortality and morbidity. This problem was not considered to be due to the lack of physicians, nurses, other health personnel, facilities, and modern technology, as I had anticipated.

In many societies local customs practiced during or shortly after the delivery of infants are responsible for causing neonatal tetanus. In Eastern cultures, for example, the umbilicus may be cut ritualistically by a bamboo knife. In other cultures the severed umbilicus is covered with mud or cow dung. In some nomad tribes in the Mid-East the infant is swathed or blanketed in fresh, warm cow or camel dung, which is to keep the infant warm and stimulate the circulation. They believe this practice serves an important physiological and possibly lifesaving function. In all these examples tetanus frequently results since this organism is almost always present in bovine feces and river mud. Another example of potentially life-threatening cultural practices was seen when female infants' ears were routinely pierced by the mothers. For the female child, pierced ears and jewelry are related to early, arranged marriages and thus to the mothers' concerns for the welfare and security of their daughters. Nevertheless, tetanus and death often resulted.

A ten-month-old child who had scurvy and a very swollen and enlarged knee was breast-fed by his malnourished mother, his only source of food. She treated the swollen joint by the folk practice of vigorous rubbing, not unlike a layman's approach to such a situation in any country. In this case there was hemorrhage into the knee joint.

Other more elaborate and ritualistic practices used by families not only complicate the illness but also cause additional disease. An infant born at home who developed tetanus was treated with lead pigment by painting the skin on the forehead, the nostrils, and palms of the hands. These were sites the parents could identify as problem areas, since he had convulsions, flaring nasal alae, and spasms producing clenched fists. They also fed him the lead in butter that produced, in addition to his other problems, acute lead poisoning.

In developing nations even the medicine that comes from new technological developments can have a negative effect when not used properly. The parents of an eleven-month-old female, in an attempt to assure her health, bought what they thought were vitamins but what was actually a hormone preparation. The child developed precocious secondary sex characteristics and vaginal bleeding.

Many folk medical practices may be harmless in that they do not produce disease or complications of an existing disease, but these practices may be considered cruel or inhumane by the out-group or the uninitiated. One of the most frequent practices used by the Bedouins in Saudi Arabia, for example, is cautery. Used for thousands of years as a means of warding off evil and combating certain types of diseases, cautery is successfully used in pain and muscle spasms. The counter-irritant theory of pain gives a plausible scientific basis for its success, for those who need to have a scientific basis. It may also be used for a variety of other conditions such as asthma, colic in infants, and gastroenteritis. It is used when all else has failed, as a last resort. Where there is a feeling of despair people are willing to turn to practices based on superstition, not sanctioned by religion—in this case Islam. One newborn infant was treated by cautery around the umbilicus and had small circular burns surrounding the umbilicus. The baby had tetanus, and the parents in some way correctly associated the umbilicus with the disease and cauterized the area. More extensive cautery was used in a four-year-old male who had longstanding malnutrition and gastroenteritis. The cautery was used where the problem seemed to be, on the abdomen, which was distended, and on the chest, because he was in respiratory distress secondary to dehydration and electrolyte imbalance. The extensive burns from the cautery were second and third degree.

A much less disturbing form of treatment, not only to us but to the patient, was given to an infant whose anterior fontanel was depressed, secondary to diarrhea and dehydration. A poultice of egg and flour was applied to the affected region and henna dye was used as part of a ritual to treat this infant.

None of these infants and children lacked attention by their parents; all were highly valued by their parents. When the children were in the hospital the fathers and mothers were very involved and proud of their children. One mother, veiled as usual from head to toe, eagerly would feed her infant the foods she was taught to prepare in the hospital, using foods that were locally available to her.

For the treatment of universal illnesses or self-limiting conditions such as colic and umbilical hernia, folk practices are nearly unlimited. Some people bind the abdomen. In Hawaii a red marker was put on the head and the abdomen was massaged because the stomach was thought to be reversed or upside down. Many cultures place a metal coin over the umbilicus. Such practices may have therapeutic value even though they have secondary complications such as fungus infection developing under the coin.

Whether the practice is harmless, harmful, or just offensive to the staff's values of what is "right" is an important differentiation that a health professional has to make. One of the differences frequently pointed out between traditional cultures and the people of industrialized nations is the resistance of the former to change. This stereotypical approach also suggests that an industrialized society takes precautions through its government, sets up a series of safeguards to protect the patient and, by using a scientific approach, readily discards treatment that does not meet the established therapeutic standards or that is potentially damaging to the patient. Furthermore, people in industrialized nations believe that treatment not thoroughly safe is not used. The following examples point to the danger of such stereotypical thinking:

1. In the 1950s, as part of the push by certain interests to increase bottle feeding of infants, a new liquid formula was marketed with great enthusiasm; it was given away in hospitals and doctors' offices. Because Vitamin B_6, pyrodoxine, was inactivated during the sterilization process, many infants had convulsions(9, 10).

2. A liquid soap routinely used in hospital nurseries throughout the United States virtually eliminated staphylococcus infections in the nurseries. At the same time, however, it caused the death of some infants because it was absorbed through the skin in sufficient levels to be toxic(11, 12).

3. One of the new broad-spectrum wonder drugs in the 1950s cured many infants and children of infectious diseases. Nurses noted, however, that premature infants on the drug turned gray and rapidly died. The premature infant's liver could not detoxify excessive dosages of this drug, and premature kidneys could not eliminate it(13, 14).

4. Another new wonder drug in the 1950s was, and still is, a sure cure for many bacterial infections. It was considered an ideal drug to use in combination with other drugs for the treatment of pulmonary tuberculosis, meningitis due to influenza, and to be used prophylactically in many newborn nurseries. That is, until it was discovered that it produced damage to the eighth cranial nerve, vestibular damage, and auditory damage with permanent hearing loss. These autotoxic characteristics may also produce damage to the fetus in utero when given to the pregnant woman(15).

5. An infamous and pathetic example of a disease contracted through our attempts to save lives and prevent disease is retrolental fibroplasia. Premature infants who would have died without a high percentage of ambient oxygen in their incubator became blind from the effects of excessive oxygen(16).

6. A more recent example is the advent of an epidemic in the United States of the Guillain-Barre Syndrome (GBS) resulting from a swine flu bivalent influenza vaccine mass immunization program in 1977. There were 354 reported cases of GBS and at least fourteen deaths(17). The controversy still exists about the

real danger of a swine flu influenza epidemic in 1977. There is no doubt, however, that many scientists believed that they were protecting the lives of children and families.

There are more such instances in the medical archives in the not-so-distant past. All these examples represent a sincere commitment and concern for bettering the lives of infants and children when, in fact, these efforts have damaged many of them.

These events in this highly technological industrialized society are very similar to the practices of different cultures whose folk medical practices do not fit our current concepts of appropriate medical care. The concern and commitment is similar, if not identical, to that seen in the parents of infants and children in the developing nations and in various ethnic groups in the United States. All these parents did and still do what they can to fight disease to save their children's lives. What appear to be cultural differences in health-seeking behaviors and health-providing behaviors may be in fact manifestations of the same motivations, but on different levels with different degrees of scientific background.

With little effort we can find examples showing that we, in the health professions in this country, are bound to rituals. Some rituals come close to being superstitious practices, although we are motivated by our concern and commitment to infants and children. As seen by the examples given, several of these practices have in the past proven to be damaging and even disastrous. The resistance to viewing these with critical scientific criteria has been phenomenal and much more characteristic of the theoretically traditional society than of an advanced technological society. A knowledge of class and cultural characteristics and differences is a beginning in the understanding of health care of both the seeker and the provider.

We need to take the next steps beyond awareness of the cultural patterns and understand the individualistic needs on which they are based. We need to understand how these underlying universal values may be used to provide optimum health care rather than allowing a cultural practice, whether it is unfamiliar to us or one of our own "sacred cows," to act as a barrier to health care.

REFERENCES

1. Herzog, E., & Lewis, H. Children in poor families: Myths and realities. *American Journal of Orthopsychiatry*, 1970, *40*, 375–387.
2. Stewart, J. C., Jr., Lauderdale, M., & Shuttlesworth, G. E. The poor and the motivation fallacy. *Social Work,* November 1972, *17*, 34–37.
3. Statistical Report. Honolulu: State of Hawaii, Department of Health, 1977.
4. EPHI, *The child growth & development inventory.* Honolulu: University of Hawaii, School of Public Health, 1975. Unpublished document.
5. Bass, M. A., & Wakefield, L. *Community nutrition and individual food behavior.* Minneapolis: Burgess, 1979.
6. Lowenberg, M. E. *Food and people.* New York: Wiley, 1979. Third Edition.
7. Aamodt, A. M. Culture. In A. L. Clark (Ed.), *Culture, childbearing, health professionals.* Philadelphia: Davis, 1978.
8. Arnold, F., Bulatao, R. A., Buripakdi, C., et al. *The value of children: A cross-national study. Vol. I. Introduction and comparative analysis.* Honolulu: East-West Population Institute, 1975.
9. Malon, C., & Parmelee, A. Convulsions in young infants as a result of pyridoxine (vitamin B_6) deficiency. *Journal of the American Medical Association,* 1954, *154*, 405–426.
10. Coursin, D. Convulsive seizures in infants with pyridoxine deficient diet. *Journal of the American Medical Association,* 1954, *154*, 406–408.
11. Kimbrough, R. Review of toxicity of hexachlorophine. *Archives of Environmental Health,* August 1971, *23*, 119–122.
12. *Physician's Desk Reference.* Oradell, NJ: Medical Economics Company, 1979, pp. 1057–1058.
13. Sutherland, J. Fatal cardiovascular collapse of infants receiving large amounts of chloramphenicol. *American Journal of Diseases of Children,* June 1959, *97*, 761–767.
14. Burns, L., Hodgman, J., & Cass, A. Fatal circulatory collapse in premature infants receiving chloramphenicol. *New England Journal of Medicine,* December 1959, *261*, 1318–1321.
15. Robinson, G., & Cambon, K. Hearing loss in infants of tuberculous mothers treated with streptomycin during pregnancy. *New England Journal of Medicine,* 1964, *271*, 949–951.
16. James, S., & Lanman, J. T. (Eds.) History of oxygen therapy and retrolental fibroplasia. *Pediatrics,* Supplement, 1976, *57*, 591–634.
17. U. S. Department of Health, Education and Welfare, Center for Disease Control. *Morbidity and Mortality Weekly Report,* February 11, 1977, *26*, 41–52.

part **II**

INTERVENTIONS FOR THE FAMILY IN HEALTH CARE

unit C
FAMILY-CENTERED UNITS

10

ecology of care

MARVIN ACK

Marvin Ack, PhD, is Director of Mental Health/Ecology at the Children's Health Center, Minneapolis, Minnesota. As part of an administrative group committed to a quality mental health environment, Dr. Ack describes an approach that is designed to enhance family strength.

Ecology concerns itself with the relationship between organisms and their environment. Any institution that seeks to have a successful program must fully understand the nature and needs of the organism at various stages of development, as well as knowing which aspect of the institution will be most helpful. People and hospitals are dynamic entities and there are no absolutes. What can be helpful at one moment can be difficult and painful at another. Let me give you some examples of situations in which the thoughtless application of what would usually be useful behaviors may have created some problems.

John, thirteen years of age, entered the hospital for a relatively routine surgical procedure. This hospital admission was his first and the first for anyone in the family other than for birth. He was very anxious, and his parents were quite protective. A member of the hospital staff recommended to his mother that she might want to spend the night with her son. Following the operation John behaved in a very immature infantile fashion.

Was his regression an expected reaction to illness, hospitalization, and surgery, or could that behavior have been brought about by the prophecy of the staff person and the parent whose behavior toward John said, in effect, "We don't think that you are going to be able to manage this on your own."

Heather is five years old, and she was scheduled for a tonsillectomy. The hospital to which she was going had pre-hospitalization and pre-surgical tours, but they had them only every other week because of a shortage of staff and a shortage of volunteers. Therefore, Heather actually heard all the intimate details of her hospitalization and her pending surgery almost four weeks before the experience. When she came to the hospital to become a patient she was almost in a panic state; she had rather conscious concerns and fantasies of being destroyed. Her parents handled these statements by ridicule, saying, "Oh, come on. You were on the tour, and you know that's foolish. Nothing like that is going to happen." Needless to say, Heather was almost impossible to anesthetize and then very difficult to manage on the ward. There is a very high correlation between children who are difficult to anesthetize and their later behavior on the ward.

Was this girl's disorganization a characteristic product of her personality under stress, or could it have been the result of having to live for three weeks with the intimate knowledge of impending surgery?

Kevin is a seven-year-old who fractured a limb in a bicycle accident and was rushed to the emergency room. On his way to the hospital he mustered up all the images of masculinity that he could, and he presented himself as a rather stoic soldier. The resident physician, having heard that preparation is important, immediately informed Kevin of exactly what was going to be done.

Despite the fact that he did this in a very reassuring tone, following the information Kevin seemed to decompensate and began to fight the nurses and the rest of the staff.

Was this obstreperous behavior the result of coming into contact with the reality of the hospital, or might it have been precipitated by the comprehensive explanation he received immediately before the procedures? These last two examples ask the questions: Is there an optimum time for preparation? Can information be given too early or too late, to the detriment of the patient? Can an ecology program be planned without a theory of anxiety? These brief vignettes are offered to suggest that a simplistic idealism is not a sufficient foundation for an ecology program. Such a hospital-wide program must be based on a solid scientific foundation. Where demonstrable fact or research evidence is not available, a comprehensive, useful theory of psychological functioning must guide our behavior. Unless we have data or theory to substantiate or guide us, we are reduced to an unacceptable ascientific, atheoretical pragmatism. Since we are frequently accused by our medical colleagues of, at worst, practicing black magic or, at best, offering little more than common sense, we must not fuel these criticisms by any sort of thoughtlessness. I have heard words such as *caring, loving, humanism,* and *humanitarianism.* There is no question that this is all absolutely necessary, but this is not sufficient.

I shall now present some of the philosophical, theoretical, and scientific premises that underlie our efforts at the Children's Health Center in Minneapolis. I am not going to claim that everything we do is correct or that it always works out well. However, I will claim that what we do in this area is thoughtful. Our programs and their contents are determined either by research data or by theoretical propositions.

BIOPSYCHOSOCIAL ASSUMPTIONS

We began with the assumption that all illness is psychological, social, and organic. This biopsychosocial approach says that all hospital personnel who purposefully come in contact with patients are engaged in treating disease and promoting health. If you accept such a model it does away with an arbitrary mind/body dichotomy. It even does away with the entire category of psychosomatic medicine. The belief in the category labeled *psychosomatic* provides the organically-minded physician or nurse with a convenient excuse to ignore certain patients by simply turning them over to a department of psychiatry or, worse, telling the patient it is all in his head. Somehow such a pronouncement is supposed to make the pain or worry less intense.

The acceptance of this biopsychosocial model elevates all persons dealing with the nonorganic aspects of illness to a level of equal partnership with the physician. (Unfortunately that is not true in salaries, but it is true in the way we treat patients.) On a practical level this biopsychosocial model demands that all persons dealing with a patient or his family, such as chaplains, child life persons, or social workers, chart their findings and that all patient care conferences involve these people. Such a conceptualization tells the admitting department that the attitude of the family and the patient toward the hospital and its efforts may be determined by the quality of that first contact. Such a conceptualization says to the doctor that the way in which a diagnosis is made may be just as important as the accuracy of that diagnosis. There are many other practical implications of this point of view.

Our next assumption is that the science of child development underlies the efforts of all the disciplines dealing with children. Our entire inservice training program as well as our staff consultative efforts are shaped by this belief. Our articulated position vis-à-vis our colleagues is that an appreciation of our knowledge of child development can make a better professional and make the job easier.

TRAINING FOR STAFF

Our ecology staff does not try to make mental health workers of doctors or nurses. We simply try to make these people better doctors or nurses by helping them become more sensitive to and more knowledgeable about the children with whom they work. From a practical perspective, everyone in the hospital receives training in the appropriate aspects of child psychology, child development, or child psychopathology. The biopsychosocial approach demands that every department in the hospital have an ecology consultant to whom they can go when issues arise that seem unresolvable. I hope you understand the full impact of this program. Literally everyone who works in our hospital will sometime or other go through a training program in child psychology taught by some member of the ecology staff, a psychiatrist, a psychologist, a social worker, or someone who is capable of teaching that subject. In addition, every department will have a consultant to whom they can go when issues arise. Since the range of human problems is infinite, it is not likely that the limited insight that professionals not trained in mental health get from their own training or even from our didactic efforts will be sufficient to meet all contingencies. The types of problems that I am referring to may concern patient care but also may include intrastaff problems or even unrecognized systemic difficulties. The departments with consultants go beyond patient care services to include housekeeping, maintenance, food service, admitting, and so forth. Not only do almost all the employees go through a training program in psychology, not only does each department have a consultant, but also every other Thursday we have mental health grand rounds to which everyone in the hospital is invited. Every week we have pediatric grand rounds, and one of those meetings every two months must have a mental health topic. Thus, we make certain that the doctors always hear some of what is labeled the psychological aspects of physical illness. In addition, one of the quarterly staff meetings for the attending staff must have a mental health topic. We constantly inundate the staff with mental health issues, their importance, and their effect on the patient's care and recuperation. These conferences allow us to demonstrate what a comprehensive psychological study can or cannot accomplish; we find that we must guard against unrealistic magical expectations that others may have of us.

THE ECOLOGY CONCEPTS

The overall purpose of our ecology program is not simply to lessen the traumatic effect of hospitalization, but rather to develop and maintain an environment where growth can take place and ultimately where health is promoted. Health is much more than the absence of disease.

If the two propositions that I have presented to you underlie our reason for being, what are the concepts that dictate our everyday functioning? We began with the psychoanalytic definition of a trauma. This concept of trauma as the precipitating agent producing emotional problems was valuable in helping us determine preventive procedures. Trauma is an overwhelming experience that a person cannot understand and for which he is not prepared. A trauma creates a distortion in development. We reasoned that if our individual behavior and our collective institutional behavior reversed these elements, we could reduce traumas to simply difficult life circumstances. These life circumstances, if mastered, encourage personality organization and promote growth. There is no reason to be concerned about the fact that a person has to experience a difficult circumstance, because those experiences can produce growth if the person masters it. What a person cannot master tends to be overwhelming. The practical consequence of this is to try never to overwhelm children. We do not restrain children for injections; we do not make walking rounds where a doctor and five residents poke the painful part of a child and then discuss their findings in somber tones in the child's presence. We also know that extremes tend to promote emotional difficulties so, as much as possible, we do things gradually. We try to prepare children for all procedures and recognize that preparation is much more than simply telling a child the facts. All of our personnel have learned to understand the role of fantasies and most of them will attempt to elicit and to work through pathognomic fantasies before telling the child any real fact. By now, nurses on our staff who work with cardiac patients are as skilled as our mental health staff at eliciting and dealing with anxiety-producing fantasies. Volunteers for our weekly pre-operative program take the children for a tour through the hospital and then spend an additional hour with children playing and trying to bring hidden, disturbing ideas to consciousness. These volunteers have had biweekly training sessions with me over a period of a year. They are very astute. They know enough to recognize children whose problems go far beyond the immediate situation and beyond their capabilities. In those instances the volunteers give the child's name and their observations to the head nurse of the unit where the child is going. This notice prepares the nurse and the staff for the child's arrival. If the head nurse then determines that the behavior is beyond their capacity, an ecology worker will be notified and will begin to work with the patient, the family, or both at no additional cost to the patient.

To assist us more specifically, we supplemented this program with preventive behavior, both individual and institutional, that was developed from our understanding of the psychoanalytic theory of anxiety and its stages. We know, for example, that anxiety can be debilitating but also can be adaptive. Too much anxiety can overwhelm a person and produce a crisis. A modicum of anxiety serves as a signal to the ego to erect defenses and thereby prepare the person for an impending danger. We are just as concerned about the child who comes into the hospital without any apparent anxiety as the child who comes in a panic. The rigidly defended child may appear to be without concern, but if anything untoward occurs he has no mechanism available for adaptation. Most studies indicate that the people who do poorest in hospitals are those at either extreme; that is, those who come in without any anxiety whatsoever or those people who come in a panic, fearful that they are going to die. The knowledge of the stages of anxiety was very helpful in determining rules and initiating programs.

WORKING TOGETHER WITH PARENTS

We know that the major source of anxiety for the very young child is the separation from his parents, which often produces a fear of abandonment. Therefore, when such a child comes into the hospital we urge parents to stay, and we make provisions for them to do so. We encourage the parents to accompany their children through all procedures, through x-ray and anesthesia, and to hold the child. Parents even hold the child on their lap when the anesthesiologist administers anesthesia to the child. When we have parents who, for whatever reason, cannot stay, we have a "Bedside Buddy" program. In this program a volunteer will stay with the child each day, usually for the entire length of his internment. The volunteer may agree to stay a week or ten days and may not come again for four more weeks or until her turn comes up again. We will have the same person serve as one child's "Buddy" throughout the stay. We do have primary nursing, but even then it is hard to give the small child the intense involvement that is needed.

If we have an eight- or nine-year-old, however, we do not encourage the parents to spend the night. The average child this age will feel uncomfortable without his parents, but he knows that he will not be abandoned. Having his parents stay might easily be seen as infantilizing or as an invitation to regress. If the child can comfortably manage the separation, he will more than likely feel very proud of his capacity to deal with events in a mature and in an age-appropriate fashion. I know there are some new hospitals that have an adult bed for every child bed, but it would not be in the adolescents' best interest, for example, to have their parents stay with them. That is what I mean by the thoughtless application of what is generally a good idea.

Another of our beliefs is that the family and friends are an integral part of the child's healing process. As a consequence we encourage parents and friends to visit as much as they can for as long as they wish. If the parents are anxious or concerned, we offer them psychological services, again at no additional cost. Twice a week we have meetings for parents who have children on the ward to help them aid their child's adjustment to the hospital and its procedures and the illness. Our social worker simply says that we are going to have a meeting for the next hour, that we will serve coffee and donuts, and would the parents like to join us? Either the social worker, the chaplain, or some other skilled person will work with the parents. "How is your child doing? Is he anxious. What's happening?" This constant concern makes the parents feel cared about. We also attempt to foster adaptation by offering the patient and family as much control over their circumstances as is medically warranted. For example, to the youngster who comes into the emergency room we might say, "Would you prefer to have your parents with you or would you like them to wait outside?" "Do you want me to tell you the things I am going to do, or would you rather that I just simply go ahead and do them and we can talk about them later?" "Would you like the shot in the right arm or the left arm?" It is not much of a choice, but it is something.

Parents are encouraged to take over as much of the nonmedical care of their child as they wish and to assist nurses in other duties. We urge the patient to take on as much activity as is reasonable. We offer as much information as the child can appreciate and integrate. For example, we will frequently take latency age patients to the laboratory so that they can see blood samples analyzed and to radiology to show them x-ray films. In this fashion we encourage an appropriate use of intellectualization, not as a defense but rather as a coping mechanism. We foster the sense of control by giving the patient and family as much responsibility over their care as is reasonable.

STAFF SUPPORT

This theory of anxiety is as helpful in our ecological work with our staff as it is with direct patient care, since the anxiety over loss is almost as great for adults as it is for children. We have support groups for nurses and others on a regular basis. We also have ad hoc groups whenever we have an unusually stressful time. If, for example, in our intensive care unit, three or four children die, that is really hard for the staff to deal with, so we have a support group. We have a very low nursing turnover rate in our intensive care unit, about two percent per annum over the last six years, even in the most stressful period. The reason for this is that we have many types of services for those nurses. They love working there, and they do not leave. We sometimes notice that separation anxiety or anxiety over loss occurs among the staff when a long-term patient has recovered, not only when someone has died. When a patient you have taken care of and loved has to leave, it can be a very debilitating and difficult experience. We have had to help our staff deal with anxiety arising from fear of loss of control of their own sexual or aggressive impulses because, occasionally, chronically ill or handicapped patients, angry at fate, displace this anger onto the staff, and the staff is tempted to respond in kind. However those hostile wishes are so at odds with the patient's own self concept that sometimes enormous anxiety gets aroused. At times we have had adolescents whose concern about their physical adequacy has led to an increase in overt sexual activity. This activity can take the form of masturbation or inappropriate behavior with nurses or with other patients. These behaviors may arouse similar anxiety among the staff, many of whom are themselves only recently out of adolescence. The ecology consultant can help the staff deal with this anxiety and help the staff avoid expressing themselves inappropriately with patients.

WORKING THE SYSTEM

There are as many helpful approaches and behaviors as there are people. A person cannot dictate staff's specific acts, since each person has to function in a way that is personally comfortable. I am very opposed to the consultant who says that there is only a single way to deal with any given patient. However, each person on our staff must know that adaptation is fostered by knowledge, by activity, by responsibility, and by control.

We pride ourselves in feeling that we have an open system, characterized by dynamic and fluctuating features. We consider everyone who works in the hospital an ecology worker. We also have a formal organization, an ecology council. This council consists of an anesthesiologist, a radiologist, a pathologist, two pediatricians, and the director of nursing. The ecology council meets monthly to examine hospital rules and programs that need ecological consideration. Each of the people on this council is uniquely qualified to help us understand the intimate aspects of hospital functioning that an observer or a consultant may never divine on his own. The group also helps us to look at traditional health care delivery methods to see which ones might be profitably changed. For example, if there is a pediatric group with seven members, so that each day there is a different person making hospital rounds, what does that do to the patient? Or, how many times has the resident written orders so the laboratory technician has to take four and five samples of blood instead of taking it on one occasion? But sometimes it is only these people who can tell what is happening. A person cannot simply go into a hospital and assume to know how to change the system.

In addition to the hospital-based Ecology Council, we also have a Mental Health Advisory Committee. This is a committee of the Board of Trustees and is made up of twelve community professionals; there are three psychiatrists, three psychologists, three social workers, one pediatrician, and two nonmedically-related professionals. The committee meets monthly to oversee the Hospital Ecology Program. They are qualified to keep us abreast of community needs and attitudes. So you see, with a Hospital Ecology Council and a Mental Health Advisory Committee, we have a lot of people helping with their intellect, their insight, and their concerns.

11

mothers in neonatal intensive care

DONALD H. GARROW

Donald H. Garrow, BM, FRCP, is Consultant Pediatrician for the Special Care Baby Unit at Wycombe General Hospital in High Wycombe, Bucks, England. He tells about a parent living-in program in an infant intensive care unit and describes the joys and frustrations of working with parents of sick newborns.

A special care baby unit that we have in England seems to be unique in having facilities built into it for so many mothers. There is not, in England at any rate, another special care baby unit that caters to mothers on such a lavish scale.

The unit is small, not a regional center, in High Wycombe's district general hospital that serves a population of about a quarter of a million people. Of the 2,500 to 3,000 deliveries a year about 250 babies a year are admitted to the unit. More than seventy percent of the mothers of these babies are admitted with them.

In the children's ward there are twenty beds in eight cubicles

135

for resident mothers and there is free visiting. This is in accordance with our now recommended national policy. Parents may also sleep by their children's sides in the main part of the ward. Parents are part of the scene, and junior medical staff become accustomed to working with them in an arrangement that seems natural, homelike, and helpful.

This good practice, which is familiar to you I suppose, is beginning to interest the less civilized areas of Europe where mothers are not admitted with their children. It started more than twenty-five years ago in Amersham, a town seven miles away, at Amersham General Hospital. My colleague, Dr. Dermod MacCarthy, started letting mothers stay with their children, not only with their babies if they were breast-feeding or desperately ill, but with any of their children admitted to the hospital. This practice has spread to the rest of the country and, although there are areas of imperception, it is generally seen to be good.

It is strange that only in the past few decades, thanks largely to the work of John Bowlby(1, 2) and the Robertsons(3, 4) in England, Marshall Klaus and John Kennell(5) in the United States, and Peter de Chateaux(6) in Sweden, among others, that it has been recognized that newborn babies and their mothers in sickness and in health need each other. The Wycombe Special Care Baby Unit was built to avoid the separation that admission of the baby so often entails, and it enables mothers to participate in the care of their babies as far as possible.

The mother delivers the baby in the labor ward and, if her baby needs to come along to the special care unit, she will come too, with the baby in her arms. (A slide is shown of a mother who has come from the labor ward with her baby in her arms. She has an intravenous infusion.) It seems practically impossible nowadays to have a baby without having a drip [intravenous] in the back of a hand, which is tiresome for holding babies and cuddling them.

Mothers can have their babies by their beds and bring them into their bed to sleep all night if they wish. Babies room-in day and night.

In the intensive care unit, the warm nursery, about twenty to twenty-five infants are on respirators each year. We cannot manage more than two at a time. We worry that we may not have enough practice to be as good as a regional center, but I emphasize that we practice intensive care to underline that it is possible to combine the homelike atmosphere, which having mothers living-in provides, with the care of very ill babies. One mother of twins delivered tiny babies at twenty-seven weeks gestation and was with us for six weeks doing a great deal for them. The father was there, also. One of the twins died after four weeks; the other is alive and well. It was a very harrowing struggle but she has testified on a radio program about our unit and what a help it was to have been involved throughout.

Parents get quite good at practical procedures. Being involved takes the fear away from what may otherwise seem like a gruesome picture.

Should fathers be around? Should husbands be allowed to sleep in the unit with their wives? We do have fathers sleeping in with their wives, although this shocked at least one of my obstetrical colleagues and some members of the senior nursing staff who have great fears for the junior nurses discovering some of the facts of life. One gets the impression that fathers now do take a more active and responsible role in the bringing up of their children than they did in my day. The man after all, is just as capable of parental feelings as the woman. Times have changed. I remember when I was a medical student, I wanted to see what went on when breast-feeding took place. I went into the maternity ward and the Sister [nurse] in charge said, "Get out of there! You're a man, you'll curdle the milk!" But in our unit fathers are welcome. (A slide is shown of a father watching his wife feeding their baby.) He may be curdling the milk and goodness knows what he may do next.

QUESTION: I noticed on your slides a mother who was reaching into the incubator still had on her watch and her ring.

GARROW: I think I should take my watch off and wash my hands and perhaps you and the rest of us should, but it is less important for the mother to do this. She is told to wash and scrub, but she forgets, as I do. We have not had any problem with cross-infection in spite of having siblings as well as grandparents and friends. I try to persuade people not to handle babies unnecessarily and not to do things unnecessarily. I tend, for instance, not to wash before I handle the first baby. I consider it good enough if I am socially clean. But after seeing the first baby if I am going to touch another one, I wash. I do not think a person should overscrub. You just get sore places and infections on your hands. I did not notice that she was wearing a ring and I am rather glad. I do not think rings have ever been shown to carry infection. Equipment is more worrying than rings. Incubators are terrible. I am trying to get rid of them. They are a waste of money and I think they are clumsy, horrible, inhuman things.

QUESTION: Would you comment on sibling visiting? You showed a mother, a father, a new baby, and a sibling all sitting on the bed. I loved it. I am working very hard to implement that at my hospital, but it seems that everybody has a set of values to place on this. We have been allowing sibling visiting on what I call an exceptional basis. If the parent asks, then we do it. We have not had any increase in infections, but our pediatricians and our Infection Control Committee are just berserk. The only people who are really for it are the obstetricians.

GARROW: This is very extraordinary because it is usually the other way round. I had an eight-year struggle, such as you seem to be having, trying to persuade my obstetrical and midwifery colleagues to allow siblings to visit their mothers who were in the hospital having had a baby.

Children now can do this. They see the babies on respirators or whatever else, and they take it in their stride. They are not upset. All we ask is that people with colds or any infection keep away. They are very conscientious and good about it. We do not wear masks, caps, gowns, or overshoes. I tend to take my coat off because it is so hot. It is ridiculous to ask parents to dress up in what I consider an absurd way when they see me coming in without those things.

QUESTION: In our unit we are very inconsistent. We have gone in for the birthing room concept, and we allow siblings in the birthing room and siblings in the recovery room for normal delivery and then we tell them, "But you have to wash and gown if you want to see the baby on the unit."

GARROW: These practices are very mysterious. They have nothing to do with infection. It is just part of the mumbo-jumbo of the civilized world. I am ashamed and horrified that there are pediatricians doing this; I can forgive obstetricians and surgeons because they spend so much of their time dressing up. Pediatricians have no excuse.

QUESTION: That is what we are trying to deal with. What happens is that some of the pediatricians will say, "Well, I am not against it personally, but. . . ."

GARROW: May I suggest that the way to effect a change is to ask for the change to be made for a trial period? This has a better chance of being accepted and, if it works, the trial period can be indefinitely extended. When it can be seen how expertly a mother can care for her own sick baby no one will come along and say, "We must put an end to this kind of thing. I don't think we can have this anymore."

COMMENT: We have a twelve-bed unit where we do not have rooming-in until the baby is ready to go home. Then we have care-by-parent for two or three days, sometimes extended if they are not quite ready to try it on their own. Throughout the time, the parents have unlimited twenty-four hour visiting. It has not caused any kind of congestion at all. In fact they are encouraged to come in even if they want to spend hours and hours during the night.

COMMENT: We have a twelve-bed intensive care unit and then a twelve-bed step-down unit for intermediate care. We allow parents unlimited privileges, grandparents and siblings on an exceptional basis depending on the situation, but we have a center where most of our babies come in from areas outside the city. They are transported in because we are the regional center. In the step-down unit we have care-by-parents and rooming-in. I was wondering how long the mothers can stay in the rooming-in if you have a child who is going to be there for an extended period.

GARROW: They can stay as long as they like and this is where the admission of fathers becomes important. The mother of a firstborn baby who may be in for several months will, after a week or two, become torn between her loyalty to the baby to whom she is beginning to get hooked and to her husband who is alone at home. If he is admitted he will feel less out on a limb and he can share the experience his wife is having and give her support. Soon after we opened, a mother stayed a couple of weeks. Then she went home to join her husband; within a week she came back because she felt she wanted to. This is good because it indicated that the facility was appreciated. We should have offered her husband a bed, but it was early days and we simply did not think of it then.

QUESTION: Can the mother live in like that if the baby is absolutely too small to be moved out of the bed or if it is on a respirator?

GARROW: She stays in as long as she likes.

QUESTION: I am thinking of a two-pounder that you might be hesitant to move out of the main nursery.

GARROW: Oh, yes. Any of the mothers can freely move into the intensive care area. There are no restrictions. In that case the baby may be unable to come to her, but we have tried experiments using the mother as an incubator. She is a most efficient machine for raising body temperature. We have put 1,500 gram babies between a mother's breasts. The babies have become warm quicker than in an incubator. The mothers have appreciated this. They like to feel their babies.

QUESTION: Are you collecting data on your program?

GARROW: Yes, I am collecting data on four groups of babies: a group of twenty normal full-term babies who were together with their mothers in the first hour, where everything went normally and the mothers were with them every day doing everything for them, as controls. This group is compared at one month, three months, and six months of age with term and preterm babies who came to our unit with their mothers and had contact in the first hour and were involved throughout. And a fourth group of twenty babies in which there has been separation of at least two days. I am following them all at equivalent gestation ages with videotape and with very full interviews. I would hope that I can provide some evidence about the policy and facilities that we have.

QUESTION: Because nurses understand the machines and techniques that keep these babies alive they sometimes become anxious when the mother enters the picture. What can the nurse do when the mother appears not to be able to care properly for her baby?

GARROW: I am curious to understand some of the feelings of involvement and possessiveness of both staff and parents. Being physically involved in feeding and perhaps, even more, life-saving measures, makes us all feel very possessive. We have to watch out that we do not usurp the mother's role, that we do not push her out because we have, by our own involvement, become attached. We have to learn to forego the pleasure of caregiving ourselves and enjoy it vicariously through the baby's own mother. This may at first seem like a personal sacrifice and loss, but it leads to a great gain and most rewarding satisfaction. Attachment can be helped by having the babies sleeping in the rooms with the mothers and by giving more privacy and allowing them to be actually physically alone together. Our nursing staff are marvelous at not interfering. They are able just to sit and watch and not be bossy. Mothers are very sensitive in the puerperium. They may feel that they are being watched or that the nurse is feeling critical even if she is not. A mother who has not mothered before does not know whether it should be this way or that and, if she is watched, she feels awkward and it may spoil things. She must overcome her anxieties and do it her way and discover that it works. She must have a chance to be alone. Then she feels she really has a baby at last.

COMMENT: What I am faced with is that there are still a lot of feelings among nursery staff members that the babies belong to them. I just had a staff meeting with them and tried to work through the attachment concept. The obstetrical unit and the nursery are separate entities. It is so deep-rooted because twenty years ago that is what we did, mothers did not hold their babies.

COMMENT: Intensive care used to be acute care and either babies died or they got better and went home. That is not so anymore. There are many more chronically ill newborns. The nurses who have chosen to work in intensive care did not choose that kind of patient. They chose a short-term sort of thing that they do not have anymore. We are finding that we need to supply a lot more support for the nurses, because they do have to assume a nurturing role and then they grieve when a baby goes home. They say that when a baby dies, the parents have an opportunity to grieve but the nurses have another child in that bed in an hour. They do not have a chance to grieve like the parents do, although they may be in pain as well. So we have a discussion group. We do not call it therapy. If we did, no one would come. I ask one of the psychiatrists to come in for a helping session.

QUESTION: Have you seen problems such as the mother being overwhelmed with family problems or other children's needs at home and saying, "I want to go home for a couple of days; I can't take this; it's too much."?

GARROW: Yes, we do have problems, every kind of problem. But we have a social worker who comes round who keeps her ear to the ground, and the nursing staff spend a lot of time listening and talking to the mothers and getting to know them. More nurses and more time are needed to deal with this. We have not only babies to look after, but also mothers with their anxieties, apart from the fact that they may have a hemorrhage or fever. There is a continuing need to listen and then to explain. I feel quite often that women who have a baby with a fairly trivial problem get a much better deal here because the staff recognizes the need to explain everything to them and help them. With a normal baby, they may just have to get on with it because there is the next one coming off the conveyor belt.

QUESTION: You are talking about extra work for the nurses. We not only have to do some mothering of the babies but also have to mother the mother.

GARROW: Yes, but when you do that, I think then you become involved with mother and her baby. When you have a baby alone to be involved with you may resent the mother, you may feel you are the best person for that baby but, if you spend time with the mother and baby together, you know how she feels and you will find that you are helping the two of them to get along. This is different and it is a very satisfying difference.

QUESTION: How do you deal with a mother who is not interested in the baby or its care?

GARROW: She is seen not as a bad mother but as a mother who, for some reason, has not taken to her baby. It is seen as a problem, not as something to criticize. We are all interested in the mechanism of attachment, why most mothers and babies do and a few do not become attached.

QUESTION: If you have an acutely ill mother whose child is in intensive care, is she cared for in that room or does she have to remain on the other unit?

GARROW: The idea was that the mother should be able to be cared for, however ill, with her baby by her. But the obstetricians do like to keep mothers after Caesarian section. If there is a very severe toxemia, when they are still on drips and heavily sedated, they tend to stay in the postnatal ward. This is understandable. Our unit, moreover, is not ideal for giving intensive care to the mother. The intensive care is oriented to the babies. The mothers' cubicles are isolated and not immediately accessible to the nursing station. Our unit is not ideal in other ways: if you want to design such a unit, for instance, don't fail to put in a sitting room. How could I have failed to put in a sitting room? Let me explain.

I wanted the special care baby unit on the same floor as the postnatal ward. I argued that, after delivery, mothers should have their babies with them well or ill and that they should be together on the same floor. This was said to be impractical, impossible, and uneconomical, and it was not done. Somebody had been up and down the country finding it had never been done. Things had to be otherwise. The postnatal ward and well babies are upstairs, our Special Care Baby Unit downstairs on the ground floor!

I had envisaged that the mothers there would share the sitting room and facilities that the postnatal women have. This has not happened so we had to make one of our cubicles into a sitting room.

In spite of its shortcomings our unit is a good place. I think we have shown that mothers can and should be admitted to Special Care Baby Units and be involved even in the intensive care nursing of their own babies(7) .

REFERENCES

1. Bowlby, J. *Attachment and loss. Vol. I: Attachment.* New York: Basic Books, 1969.
2. Bowlby, J. *Attachment and Loss. Vol. II: Separation.* London: Hogarth Press, 1973.
3. Robertson, J. (Ed.) *Hospitals and children: A parent's eye view.* London: Victor Gollancz, 1962.
4. Robertson, J. *Young children in hospitals.* London and New York: Basic Books, 1958. London: Tavistock Publications, 1970. Second Edition.
5. Klaus, M. H., & Kennell, J. H. *Maternal-infant bonding.* St. Louis: Mosby, 1976.
6. Chateaux, P. de, Holmberg, H., Jakobsson, K., & Winberg, J. A study of the factors promoting and inhibiting lactation. *Developmental Medicine and Child Neurology,* 1977, *19,* 575–584.
7. MacFarlane, J. A., Smith, D. M., & Garrow, D. H. The relationship between mother and neonate. In S. Kitzinger & J. A. Davis, (Eds.), *The place of birth: A study of the environment in which birth takes place with special reference to home confinements.* New York: Oxford University Press, 1978, pp. 185–200.

12

once upon a time...
a father's story

MICHAEL A. LAZARUS

Michael A. Lazarus, BA, wrote this story as a compilation from parent group members who shared experiences about their newly-diagnosed infants. He and his wife celebrated their child's second birthday this year. We are indebted to Phyllis Eckert for bringing to our attention this personal story by a father.

Once upon a time there was a man and a woman who decided they would like to have a new baby, so they looked in the baby catalog to find the model they would like to have. "I would like a baby girl," said the woman. "This model will be pretty and smart, pleasant and have lots of friends. She will be number one in her class, love us very much and bring us happiness." "That sounds wonderful," said the man, "but I think I would prefer a boy baby." "He'll be very much like your model and will be successful in business. He might even make a fortune." So they thought and talked some more, and finally, later that night, sent in their order to the manufacturing plant.

In a few weeks, they were told that their order had been accepted and that production had already begun. They were both overjoyed and hurried to tell all their friends and family the good news. "There are so many things to be done," the woman said. "We have to fix up a room for the baby, buy furniture, get some clothing and some toys. Everything must be perfect." They worked and worked and soon the baby's room was beautiful. They read all the books they could find on babies. They learned all about how babies develop, and they debated about the best way to raise their new child. They read through books of names to find the one name that best suited the child they had ordered. Everything was ready.

As the months passed the reports from the inspectors at the manufacturing plant were good. "Everything seems to be going along well," they were told. "Your baby will soon be ready for delivery."

At last, the big day was here. It was time for their baby to arrive. They hurried to the delivery room at the plant. There were so many people there. Everyone was so excited. They were talking about how wonderful it would be to have a new baby at home. As the babies arrived, a technician would call out the parents' names. The excited parents rushed to see their new babies. "Oh what a lovely baby," people would say, "so pink and cute and cuddly." All the parents had big smiles and almost seemed to skip out of the room, eager to get their babies home. The man and the woman, however, were in the delivery room for quite a while. Most of the other parents were on their way home with their babies. The man and the woman began to feel a little uneasy. "Why is it taking so long?" the woman asked. "Relax," the man said, "I'm sure we will get our baby in a few minutes."

So they waited and waited until everyone else had gone and they were all alone in the room. Suddenly, one of the chief technicians came through the door. She was not smiling. "May I have a word with you?" she asked the man and the woman. "Something has gone wrong. Your baby has a problem. He is in our intensive repair unit. Come and see him."

The man and the woman did not know what to think. They followed the technician through the doors and down the corridors and through more doors and down more corridors. The woman repeated quietly, "Our baby has a problem." The man kept asking, "Intensive repair?" None of their books, or their friends, or their family had ever mentioned this! They could not understand what might have gone wrong.

When they came to the repair unit they became even more confused. They saw many technicians in odd uniforms behind the windows and strange pieces of equipment littering the room. They could hear buzzers and beepers continuously. Each sound would be followed by a flurry of activity among the technicians, who would talk loudly to one another in a language that neither the man nor the woman could understand.

Finally, among all the people and equipment, the man and the woman saw the babies who were being repaired. They both felt like they had been hit by a speeding truck. These babies were not like the ones they had seen in the delivery room. They were not pink and cute and cuddly. Some were so tiny they looked like toys. Others looked gray and lifeless. All of them had tubes and wires coming out of their bodies.

"This can't be real," said the man. "This must be a nightmare!" the woman cried. "Which one is our baby?" they asked. The technician pointed to a tiny motionless baby in the corner of the room. "Will he live?" asked the woman. "It's hard to tell," said the technician. "Your baby is in a critical situation. If he lives through the next few days, his chances will be much better, but he has a long way to go." "If he lives will he be normal?" asked the woman. The technician began to recite from a long list of manufacturing defects. The man and woman had never heard of some of the defects, some others they had heard about from telethons and other fund-raising drives. The defects were problems that happened to other people and they were not good.

As the technician droned on, the man and the woman felt more and more uncomfortable. "Why doesn't she stop?" thought the woman, "I don't want to know all this right now." Finally, when the technician was finished, the woman asked, "Which of these defects does our baby have?" "It's hard to tell," replied the technician. "Some of these defects don't show up for years. Others may develop during the next few months. We will just have to wait and see." "Why did this happen?" asked the woman, "whose fault is it?" "It's hard to tell," said the technician, reaching for the list of processing faults and material defects. "Please don't read another list," the man said. He was beginning to get angry. "You don't know if our baby will live. You don't know if he will be a normal child. You don't even know how this happened in the first place. But there's one thing I do know. This isn't the baby we ordered and we're not going to accept delivery."

"I'm sorry, sir," said the technician, "but I'm afraid you have no choice. In the Health Laws of this state it is prohibited to return or exchange babies. Why don't you wait a while and see how things turn out? You might want to speak to one of our Customer Service Workers about the situation. If you still feel the same way, she can put you in touch with our Previously-Owned-Baby Placement Service. But there is plenty of time to think about this later. Why don't you go home now and relax?"

The man and the woman walked slowly out of the plant. They thought of all the beautiful babies they had seen in the nursery. They thought of all the happy parents who were home with their babies. They thought of the beautiful room that was waiting for their baby. They thought of their family and friends who were anxiously waiting to see their new child. "What shall we tell people?" asked the woman. "Let's wait until we know more about the situation," said the man. The woman agreed and they drove home without another word being said.

13

families with newly-diagnosed handicapped infants

JESSICA G. DAVIS, PHYLLIS ECKERT, DEBORAH GOLDEN, AND SUSAN L. MCMILLAN

Jessica G. Davis, MD, directs the Child Development Center Genetics Program, and Phyllis Eckert, MSW, is a social worker with the High-Risk Pregnancy and Perinatology Programs, both of the North Shore University Hospital Cornell University College of Medicine, Manhasset, Long Island, New York. Dr. Davis proposes that families can become better prepared for genetic problems prenatally. Ms. Eckert documents episodes of unnecessary psychological trauma in parents who received the news less supportively, and suggests emotionally healthier ways to transmit information at the time the problem is identified.

Deborah Golden, MSW, is the associate director of the Children and Youth Project, and Susan L. McMillan, PhD, is a psychologist in the Child Development Division, both of the University of Texas Medical Branch in Galveston, Texas. Ms. Golden suggests ways to plan and conduct an interview to inform the family about the problem. Dr. McMillan concludes with ideas on how to build sensitivity in training health professionals about families.

PREPARING FAMILIES FOR GENETIC PROBLEMS

In order to deal with families in crisis it is necessary to remember, by understanding and examining the normal processes that occur in the parents and infant before birth, the emotional responses of a family to the birth of a child with a severe deformity. An understanding of the normal stages of development and pregnancy is also necessary in order to better appreciate a couple's response to genetic intervention.

Pregnancy is regarded as a critical period in normal biologic development. It constitutes a maturational crisis. A pregnant woman undergoes major endocrine, somatic, and psychological changes. Under normal circumstances these complex development processes prepare men and women for the task of creating a family unit, enabling both parents to undertake the appropriate parenting roles.

Until the present time little attention has been paid to the "pregnant father." Recent studies and experiences in our own unit support the notion that pregnant fathers do worry about the health and physical well-being of their yet-to-be born infants. They fantasize before their children are born and before their partner becomes pregnant. Pregnant fathers are concerned in pregnancy about their present and future relationships with their mating partner as well as with the child. They are also concerned, just as the pregnant woman is, about their future parenting responsibilities. Unfortunately, they do not speak about their feelings as often as pregnant women, and, furthermore, opportunities are rare in which such exchanges could take place if they would want to talk .

However, more and more pregnant fathers are appearing in obstetricians' offices. I think that involvement should be encouraged. Certainly fathers should become part of the developmental process of pregnancy and not be excluded or barred from office hours because of time limitations or other reasons. In our own unit we have a very good response from fathers coming for interviews. We do not make terrific demands on people; instead, we are fairly flexible in scheduling in order to include them.

Fathers-to-be are very important people, and there is a great need to better understand what they are thinking about.

Most authors believe that impregnation comes about ideally when there is an intense relationship between sexual partners. A woman's image of herself, at least according to many psychiatrists and psychotherapists, changes when she incorporates her love and her love object feelings and forms a relationship as part of her somatic being. During the first few months of pregnancy a pregnant mother's energy is increasingly focused on the foreign body, the fetus, with which she has a symbiotic relationship. The fetus becomes an integral part of herself.

At seventeen to eighteen weeks of gestation, fetal movements are first appreciated by the pregnant woman. Quickening of the fetus is experienced as the beginning of an infant's independence. It is the first time that the fetus demonstrates that it is there. This forces the parents to become aware that there is a fetus or an infant-to-be that is taking over its own destiny and that has a separate existence. Parents realize that eventually this existence will culminate in an anatomic and emotional separation during the birth process.

After eighteen weeks, the woman experiences a dual role. She nurtures the growing fetus within herself as if it were part of herself, and at the same time she experiences an increased awareness of the fetus's ability to become a separate entity. These stages, I believe, permit the groundwork to be built for a successful delivery, anatomic separation, and a relationship with that child.

Couples vary in personality, family structure, emotional adjustment, and physical strengths and weaknesses. These differences are important to consider when counseling parents. Also important is the state in which the couple entered the pregnancy, whether the pregnancy was planned or not, their life setting and developmental style, and their family constellation. For example, all pregnant women and their mates fantasize about their unborn child's appearance, personality, and future. In the early stages of pregnancy, a woman may focus her attention on the infant growing inside her; at the same time she may also experience hope for enrichment of herself, and she may dream about the child's fulfilling unmet needs or secret ambitions.

Pregnant women and their partners also have intense feelings of loss: loss of freedom, of a job, of companionship, and the impending termination of the security of their previous life style. Feelings of anger or ambivalence about these losses are not uncommon. The pregnant couple also have an understandable concern as to whether the baby will be normal, yet these concerns are rarely verbalized. Even the professionals dealing with pregnant couples do not raise the possibility of abnormality. Many professionals believe it is inappropriate to discuss because it would produce unnecessary anxiety. Many parents who have completed a pregnancy and who have a problem outcome, however, tell me that they wished that someone had given them the opportunity to air these thoughts during the pregnancy.

If a problem occurs, such as the birth of an abnormal baby at high risk for developmental disabilities, a baby with low birth weight, a baby who has experienced severe respiratory distress, or a complication of delivery, this suppressed material will surface. Parents with high-risk pregnancy outcome universally tell their physicians or counselors after the event that they did think their baby might not be normal but they never spoke about it because their thoughts were so terrifying. In addition, all such parents will tell you, as they have told me, that they believed that these problems could never happen to them. Health care providers need to offer a time and a place for these feelings to be expressed.

Having a child is tied up with ego, not only the mother's or couple's ego, but also the ego of the professional. It is shattering when things do not go well. Everyone somehow feels at fault and guilty.

Very few of the parents we see after the birth of an affected child have any knowledge of factors related to unfavorable pregnancy outcome. When I first started my work some fifteen years ago, very few couples had knowledge of genetics, embryology, or the reproductive process. Today, many couples still believe that "thinking bad thoughts" has a direct effect on the pregnancy outcome. The thought itself is believed to be the damaging agent or force that causes the problem.

Patients who are at risk for an unfavorable outcome have had a history of reproductive loss or fetal wastage, documented medical problems, or are at risk for genetic disorders. A history of reproductive loss means that the couple had two or more miscarriages or spontaneous abortions with or without a past history of having given birth to a child with some sort of genetic problem, birth defect, or congenital malformation. Often these events are coupled with the birth of a stillborn infant. Such couples have major difficulties when coming to a genetics unit or to their obstetricians for ongoing counseling. They have feelings of inadequacy, depression, and deep sorrow. These couples have marked concerns about their sexual prowess and their sexuality in general, and they believe that they are not able to function as normal men and women. Not being able to conceive a child or not being able to have a pregnancy go to term can be as devastating as having a child with a major birth defect. There are fantasies concerned with these reproductive losses that are similar to the dreamlike thoughts that occur around the birth of a malformed child.

Women with documented medical problems include those with a known medical history of hypertension, diabetes, epilepsy, or other conditions. In addition, large numbers of pregnant women request counseling and diagnostic services because of exposure to a range of potentially dangerous agents such as herbicides, medicines, and x-rays. Men with documented medical problems, including men with histories of cancer who received radiation and chemotherapy, request information about their risks. They want to learn about the potentially harmful effects of their previous medical problems and their treatment modalities on pregnancy outcome. Children who were saved from catastrophic illness now present themselves as young adults who are thinking about parenthood. In addition, publicity about possible radioactive fallout from accidents at nuclear power plants and exposure to chemical agents in the workplace result in increased demands for genetic services. And, individuals and couples come to ask about risks related to their occupations.

Patients in genetic counseling are ambivalent about their problems. Many are very anxious. Other patients deny they are at high risk for having a child with birth defects. Questions and opinions aired by these patients, however, should not be treated lightly. Their thoughts and ideas should be explored so that an appropriate kind of counseling base can be set up for each pregnant person or couple.

Many of the patients at risk for genetic disorders are healthy people who have no family history of genetic disorders or birth defects. Most have not yet had any children but they ask for counseling. Why is this happening? I think that we are seeing a great interest in genetic health and that the public has greater access to genetic information. In addition, most couples today are not thinking about having large families. Many plan to have only one or two children. These couples, therefore, want the quality of life for their children to be as ideal as possible. They want to do everything they possibly can to ensure a favorable outcome. They also come to us for reassurance that they will have a healthy baby.

Many women seek services because they are thirty-five years old or more and pregnant. They realize they are at increased risk for having a child with chromosomal problems. These patients come not only to learn about their risks but also to ask about the advances in medical technology, amniocentesis in particular.

A person or couple who have had a child with a genetic disorder also want to have testing. Conditions that call for testing in utero include a history of having given birth to a child with a chromosomal abnormality such as Down's syndrome or Turner's syndrome, an inborn error of metabolism or a biochemical problem such as Tay-Sachs disease, or a birth defect involving the neural tube or a defect of the developing nervous system, anencephaly, or spina bifida. In addition, we counsel people who are at risk of being carriers of a particular genetic trait because of their ethnic background. An example is the person with sickle cell trait, in which the person has one gene that codes for normal adult hemoglobin. Since genes work in pairs, people with that trait have a partner gene that codes for the sickle hemoglobin molecule. People with sickle cell trait have no medical symptoms from their altered gene; they can be identified only through a special laboratory test.

There are also people who, because of an unusual arrangement of their genetic material, carry a balanced chromosome abnormality. Carrier status has no effect on a person's well-being, health, or longevity but can influence the outcome of pregnancy adversely depending on how chromosomes are distributed to the person's progeny. Cytogenetic or chromosome studies are performed to identify people with rearrangements or translocation of their genetic material.

More than 40,000 women in the United States have had amniocentesis, an optional surgical procedure that is usually performed between sixteen to eighteen weeks of gestation. During amniocentesis the obstetrician withdraws about twenty cubic centimeters of amniotic fluid from the amniotic sac surrounding the fetus. The fluid is opalescent and can be analyzed for over seventy biochemical abnormalities by doing specific tests on samples of the fluid. This fluid can be monitored only for open defects of the developing nervous system. Amniotic fluid cells can be analyzed for presence of cytogenetic abnormalities.

It is the job of the geneticist to explain during a preamniocentesis counseling session what information this test can and cannot provide. The counselor must be available to answer questions, to explain the procedure, to talk about the risks involved, and to encourage the patients to talk about their fears. At this time also, the counselor obtains and reviews the family and medical histories. If at all possible, the patient and her partner are seen together. If not, the patient is encouraged to enlist the support of a family member or a close friend in order to alleviate emotional suffering or anxiety.

Because of their anxieties, patients do not remember everything that they hear the first time and are therefore encouraged to share their fears, fantasies, and concepts. We provide emotional support, availability by phone and, if necessary, follow-up visits. If a patient's obstetrician does not perform amniocentesis, the patient meets the physicians who will do the test. Patients also have time to review what they have discussed with their physicians or counselor.

In group discussions potential candidates for amniocentesis are encouraged to express their concerns about their problems and their fears about the potential pain and discomfort. Counselees have a great deal of difficulty expressing "foolish" questions while talking with physicians, nurses, or counselors and tend to bring up these concerns in this group setting instead.

Not every pregnant couple decides to undergo amniocentesis

and must not be influenced by the counselor's personal views or feelings. During the amniocentesis counseling session, the counselor presents accurate, pertinent information to the family. Often the patient needs the services of additional consultants and then reviews all the available data, weighs the risks, and makes the decision as to whether or not to have amniocentesis. Ongoing support is made available as well to those patients who decide not to undergo amniocentesis.

The third step in the program is the procedure itself. Studies have graphed levels of anxiety during the amniocentesis counseling process. There is a peak at the initial counseling session, followed by a plateau. Then a second peak occurs that lasts three weeks, because that is the time it takes for the cytogenetics results to be made available to patients. The next peak is the anxiety generated when the patient is informed of the results. If the laboratory results are normal, patients cry on the phone with relief and joy. Many call back to thank us again. If the results are abnormal, information must be exchanged about the laboratory results, the nature of the problem, or diagnosis and the prognosis. I believe this is a physician's responsibility. The medical geneticist must take responsibility for the accuracy of the laboratory tests and the sharing of critical information. These patients are not only in crisis but also are experiencing sorrow and pain. They mourn the loss of their "perfect," as yet to be born, infant. The role of the professional here is to provide sufficient, accurate information to support the family so that they can begin to adjust rationally to problems at hand and to be able to cope with all their options. The options reviewed with patients include continuation of the pregnancy with ongoing support or termination of the pregnancy with ongoing support. Patients must be helped to see that there is no wrong or right decision, that they must arrive at a "comfortable decision." Ideally, this decision must be appropriate for the person, the couple, and their family and must be compatible with their religious beliefs, their philosophy, and their life style.

IDENTIFYING THE PROBLEM

The birth of a baby with a handicapping condition, birth defect, or prematurity is an enormous trauma for parents. They react with shock, disbelief, denial, anger, grief, and guilt. This is not the baby they had planned and dreamed about. This is certainly not their "fantasy baby." Much later these parents may quip about this baby being the March of Dimes poster child, but for now, they find themselves propelled into a crisis situation. Their world has collapsed; the usual methods of coping no longer seem to work; they have lost their order of things and their equilibrium.

One father in the parents' group remembers the beginning for him in the delivery room:

> They called me in and I remember everything happening very quickly. The thing that I remember first is Dr. T. who is always in control, never gets excited; in other words, he always makes you feel he is very competent and controlled and no big problem. When the baby was born I noticed right away his whole demeanor, his whole attitude, changed. He got a very grim look on his face. He became rushed, snapping at people in the delivery room.

> He was talking, instead of in sentences and very calm, he was shouting one word things. I remember, as Judy [his wife] says, he said "Meconium." That's all he said. He didn't say anything else.

> I got the feeling that there was something wrong. And then, after the baby was born, which was a couple of minutes later, the anesthesiologist took the baby and they worked on the baby for a long time, I would say at least five minutes, before they could get the baby breathing on his own, suctioning the baby.

> I remember feeling, why isn't the baby crying, because I always waited for that picture—the baby comes out, they slap the baby or whatever, and the baby cries. Well, my baby came out—and nothing. Everyone seemed very hyper and tense and the anesthesiologist was doing a

million different things–suctioning the baby with an electric suction, with a bulb.

It is to these earliest moments that I wish to address myself, those critical moments when hospital staff can have such a powerful impact, making the difference between a nightmarish experience being ameliorated by sensitive handling or being exacerbated by the staff's own inability to cope. The staff's reactions and responses are indelibly imprinted and periodically referred to in later years.

Although there is little we can do to prevent an emergency, there are ways to handle the situation that can be helpful. Comments such as, "The baby is blue," or "He looks like he's not going to make it," or "The baby would have been better off dead," should not be said, because parents are traumatized by such comments. Saying, "I understand what you are going through," or "I know what you are feeling; I feel the same way," is inaccurate. Instead, a simple statement to the parents that this must be very difficult for them and that you will try to be available to them when they need you would be far more helpful.

Irvin, Kennell and Klaus(1) say:

> The same reactions that occur in the parents of a baby with an abnormality often occur in the nursing and medical staff, particularly the responsible physicians, in this case the obstetricians. They are performing under an unwritten promise to produce a normal infant and so may have the same difficulty as the parents in realizing that the pregnancy they have managed has resulted in the birth of a baby with an abnormality.

This guilt often is as groundless as the guilt of parents yet staff, just as parents, can feel that they might have done something more or differently. These feelings, however, can lead to an avoidance of parents, which increases their strong sense of isolation and failure.

Emotional support for parents is a known essential. However, support people change in terms of importance throughout the process. The obstetrician's role is paramount during pregnancy, delivery, and postpartum.

Support from the husband, friends, or other family members during labor and delivery has also been clearly recognized with the increasing popularity of Lamaze classes. Fathers who are present at the birth of their normal child speak of a positive, intimate involvement with the mother and baby, which is an inclusion rather than separation for the father in the family unit. It is equally important, for these same reasons, for fathers to be present at the birth of their babies if they wish to be, when problems arise. Secondary gains might include a cementing of family ties, a pulling together of husband and wife in crisis, a possible step in preventing some of the marital stress so prevalent in these families in the days, months and years to come following delivery.

One of the mothers in my group talks about the delivery room:

> They cut the cord immediately and took the baby to the other side of the room where I couldn't see her, so I turned my head and kind of bent back so I could see what they were doing and there was a whole bunch of doctors around her and they looked like they were having a lot of trouble getting her to breathe. She was very, very gray and she looked dead. I kept turning back to Bill and saying "What's wrong with the baby, the baby's not breathing, how come the baby's not breathing?" And then I realized that they weren't showing me the baby or doing any of the things that they had prepared me for like putting the baby on my stomach so that I would be able to look at her and touch her. None of those things were happening. Instead, it was just like an emergency.

> The only person I spoke with was Bill. I kept saying, "What's wrong, what's happening, what's happening?"

> They finally brought the baby over to me. They got her to breathe and they sat her on my stomach for a second. I looked at her face and she didn't look right to me and I knew her face didn't look right. And I said to Bill, "What's the matter?" and they must have given him some information because he came back a few seconds later and

said the baby was going to a special unit for observation because the baby had a stridor. I knew exactly what stridor meant and it made me very nervous and concerned. A month before, the niece of a friend of mine had a baby and she had breathing problems. She had called us up because we have medical background and asked us about stridors and we did quite a bit of research. That baby had still been in the hospital so I knew it could be very serious.

Then after Bill told me they started to roll me out of the delivery room and the anesthesiologist came over and I said, 'How's the baby?' and he said, 'Don't worry, she'll go to Harvard or Yale,' or some comment like that, like everything's fine and you have nothing to worry about. They took me to the recovery room.

At the moment he had a big smile on his face and he looked very relieved and it helped a little. But I just had a very uneasy feeling that something wasn't right. No matter what they told me, I just had that feeling. It was very strong.

When such problems occur, parents experience a precipitous drop from the original high expectations that they have brought to the delivery room. If possible, therefore, it is important for the husband to be there so that they are together during this difficult time.

The obstetrician, pediatrician, nurse, and social worker should work together in a team effort to help alleviate unnecessary stress for the family. The obstetrician, the physician with whom most parents have a strong relationship, needs to support both parents at the time of birth. Parents should be allowed to see the baby in as normal a fashion as possible under the prevailing conditions, unless they specifically request not to do so. The anxiety tends to escalate if the mother does not see the baby when it would be a normal procedure. The fantasy tends to be much worse than the reality. The obstetrician needs to acknowledge to both parents together that there may be a problem, but it is the role of the pediatrician to make the diagnosis and prognosis, if known. It is advisable for the two physicians to work together with the parents for the first two or three days until a relationship has formed with the pediatrician. The roles during this time should be carefully delineated as they develop a relationship with the new physician in an easy kind of transition.

When important information about the baby is to be shared, the mother should not be alone. She is psychologically and physically depleted. At this time she requires the support of her husband, another family member, or friend. This helps to prevent the feeling that secrets are being kept from either parent and again helps to unify the family.

Parents again and again ask for honesty, in terms that they can understand, and for compassion and time. Yet, as Kennell and Rolnick(2) point out, "No matter how intelligent or composed a parent may seem, it usually proves unwise to go into an involved explanation about tests and treatment. The family does not understand at this time or benefit from hearing about all the intricacies of medical investigations. It is easier for them and simpler for the doctor if he says initially, 'We are carrying out the necessary tests.'" If questioned further, however, the doctor should explain, simply and concisely in nonmedical language. Drawing diagrams of processes involved has proved to be helpful in facilitating concrete understanding. Parents differ in what they can handle; however, some parents need more information than others to help them feel some control over a situation that feels totally out of control. They will ask for more and the request should be respected.

In the beginning stages of the diagnostic process, parents usually know nothing of the medical situation and feel inadequate when they do not know or understand enough to respond to staff when asked, "Do you have any questions?" One father, whose son was born with a tracheo-esophageal fistula, illustrated this point when he said:

> I didn't understand what any of the doctors said for the first day and a half. Then finally I said, 'Hey, hold it. When you use something technical like that, please stop. I want the spelling of it because I want to research all of

it.' And that's the only way I got to understand what they were talking about.

The mother of a premature baby born at twenty-eight weeks gestation talked about her reactions after she left the delivery room and saw her baby in the premature nursery:

They rolled me on the stretcher back to my room with David [her husband], and on the way our doctor was telling us about his chances of survival, that we had three main worries for the first seventy-two hours: . . . sepsis, . . . respiratory distress, . . . hemorrhaging and internal bleeding. And how they could or could not handle any of those things and that the sooner the signs of any of those things occurred the closer to birth, the more serious they were. And if the baby started to slide but plateaued that was also a decent sign that it didn't have to get worse, that they could do something to help. But if the decline started and couldn't be stopped, then it would be the end. We felt that if the baby made it through the first seventy-two hours it had a decent chance. We were told that after those first three days many things were going to happen along the way but the baby could well survive because these are little things compared to the monumental things that would happen the first three days and they could be handled.

We just had no idea the rough road that we would have to travel. We got back to the room and the doctor left and David and I were talking and we just decided that we weren't going to make any calls. If anybody called me, because I was getting a lot of calls to see how I was doing, we would say, yes, the baby was born. But we weren't going to make any calls. I wasn't going to get any flowers. It was not a happy day. It was birth with reservation.

Our primary nurse came in and told us to come to the unit, call as often as we wanted, and encouraged us to be part of his care or take an active part in his development or his growth or whatever. And that was it.

We were also told that if his condition changed at all they would get in touch with us. A resident or an intern came in asking me to sign a consent form for a bilirubin light and I almost dropped dead because I thought they were coming to say that he had taken a turn for the worse. Then somebody did come in to say that they had put him on a respirator but not on full respirator, just intermittent ventilation.

I felt his chances were slim. Part of me said he's going to make it, but then when doctors and nurses started walking in and out, every time I saw somebody from the nursery I was very frightened and I really felt that this was the beginning of the end.

I also couldn't stand that he was being called male baby. It drove me crazy. Because he was so early my husband and I hadn't decided on a name. That night I just stayed up all night putting all kinds of combinations together. . . . In the morning we decided on a name. . . . I started having everybody call him by his first name because I just felt that he couldn't live or he couldn't survive without the name, just like a cat or a dog. I thought, 'Who's going to care that he couldn't survive if he wasn't personal?' I had to make him personal. That would give him life.

It is a time of much loneliness for parents, of seeing this birth as very different from a normal birth with its supports, praise, and acknowledgments. Information may have to be repeated many times in order for parents to begin to "hear." They cannot take in all the painful reality at once but only in small doses. Much psychic energy is being consumed in mourning the loss of the fantasy baby. It takes time to attempt to attach to the child for whom they never planned, the child who makes them feel like an outcast among the happy parents reveling in the miracle of birth.

Social workers can assist parents at this time, by facilitating their speaking with physicians when the parents might otherwise find much discomfort in doing so. Social workers can also evaluate parental response, help parents verbalize their feelings, and assist parents who are ready to look at the choices available to them.

Visitors bound for the maternity floor have a special look. They bear flowers, gifts, and smiles. It is the happiest area in the hospital. Tearful mothers disturb the joyful atmosphere and are not easily forgiven such transgression. It is most important, therefore, that the nurses on this floor not abandon these mothers. The role of the nurse is a particularly valuable one, from the delivery room to the nursery and postpartum floors. Communication among nurses can facilitate the continuity of the support system that was begun in the delivery room. Understanding what has happened at the birth can give the nurses on the floor a better insight into the parents' reactions and how they, as nurses, can help. Making time to listen to the mother who is reminded of her "failure" whenever the babies are brought out to feed is essential. Nursery room nurses can handle the baby with dignity and caring, and they can be accepting of the parental response. Regardless of their own feelings, parents are still observing how staff are responding to their baby. Parents should be encouraged to get involved with the care of their baby when they are able. Some parents totally reject the baby at first and that has to be respected; usually this rejection eases after one or two days.

The mother needs time to think and to talk about her feelings. It is only by being able to do so from the time of birth on that she can gradually invest feelings for her child. The father often will suppress his painful feelings in order to be supportive of his wife. Giving him an outlet to talk can be helpful. The sensitive attitudes of the professional staff at such a time are remembered quite positively. One father remarked that he had known many noncaring people during his lifetime but at the hospital total strangers had shown such concern and involvement with them that it touched him very deeply.

INFORMING THE FAMILY

Second in importance only to the early articulation of the problem is the interview with the family in which the baby's situation is discussed in depth. Families need time, space, and an opportunity to have a meaningful discussion with the care providers about what their child's situation is and will be. This interaction needs to take place after the initial period of shock has sufficiently subsided so that parents can begin to hear at least some of what is being related, to formulate questions, and to integrate the answers that they are given.

The first interpretive interview should take place before the infant's discharge or the mother's release, whichever is first. We avoid sending the mother home without giving the parents the opportunity to talk with the people who are caring for their infant. It is difficult to do this when babies are transferred from other hospitals, but we want to have a chance to see the parents before the mother goes home or the baby and mother go home together. When problems are suspected after the child is home, the child is seen as soon as possible, with the informing interview scheduled promptly thereafter. In many settings this is difficult to schedule. Evaluation clinics, for example, often have their assessment process take place over time, but anxiety and tension at home can be overwhelming for the family, so the sooner the child is scheduled the better.

The physician is the person in our projects who is primarily responsible for conducting the informing interview. We are talking about problems that originate in the medical diagnosis, so the central role of the physician is necessary and expected. We like to have primary care providers rather than specialists, if at all possible, as the core representative of the medical profession. When the neurosurgeon or the orthopedist is the core representative it creates certain problems. The active involvement of a pediatrician or family practitioner is needed. This conveys to parents that their infant is a child rather than a handicapping condition and that he or she resembles other children more than the child differs from them. The role of deliverer of well-child care and coordinator of care can also be emphasized and illustrated. Representatives of other disciplines need to be involved in the informing interview as well, since this tells parents right from the start that nurses, social workers, and others are going to have a role and are important; the physician cannot and will not do it all. It places his authority behind the value of the contributions of these people and the need for the child's and family's involvement with them.

In talking about the milieu in which the interview took place, one parent wrote of her experience:

> I had no idea what was wrong. Of course, I knew there was something but I didn't know it was anything so serious. When I went to the clinic there was a big team of them all sitting around actually laughing about some private joke. Two doctors, and then one of them said, 'Oh, well, he's blind and deaf, not much hearing here.' And there was me sitting there absolutely shattered. I can remember it so vividly. I was on my own; if I'd known there was something terrible I would have brought my husband(3).

I think this clearly reveals to us that we need the informing interview in a calm, unhurried private setting with no interruptions. Some of you are probably thinking that on your obstetrics service, there is no place to sit down. However, most postpartum women can either be wheeled or can walk to someplace where there is a little privacy and an opportunity to sit down with a staff person.

We need sufficient time at this point to be available to deal with the parents' reactions and concerns. Both parents or a supportive relative or friend should be present. Those of us who work with large populations of single mothers know that, even if the baby's father is not available, there are often other significant people who are involved. I think we must find them and try to have them there. Eventually we will have to leave the mother and baby alone, and it can be very helpful for her to have somebody there who has been through this with her. The incalculable importance of the interview to the future of both child and family demands also that we give careful attention to the atmosphere in which the interview takes place.

What is the content of this interview? What is the interchange all about? I think that depends on the child's problems, the family's concerns and their willingness to express them, and the professional's readiness to listen and respond. Sometimes the interview is a microcosm of everything that the family will ever ask or need to know. Every area is covered. However, we cannot deal with a lot of that in depth, and the families are not going to remember much of what we said. They may raise questions that are everything that they may ever bring up again, both in the immediate and distant future. There is no easy way to talk with a parent about significant disabling conditions or the high risk of one. Even if objectively we do a fairly good job, the parents' perceptions may be very different and they may broadcast their feelings and opinions widely in the community, concerning inadequacies of the information, empathy, and support provided.

In communication with parents we strive for clarity, candor, knowledge about the condition, and the nature of the help available for their child and family. We offer compassion and concern and, I think most important of all, state a readiness to admit what we do not know and what needs further investigation. We do not have to have answers to all the questions; it is important that the questions are articulated, that we let the family know it is all right to ask questions, and that we will continue to try to respond in the future as we learn more.

Some of the issues that are typically raised during the informing interview are:

- The child's chance for survival and expected life span.
- The child's capabilities, and the child's current and eventual limitations.
- The availability of treatment and/or cure including medicine, surgery, and other therapies, both standard and nonstandard.
- Effects upon family life, including cost of care.
- Whether they should maintain the child at home or should place elsewhere.
- Explaining the child's condition to others.
- The reasons for occurrence and the chance of recurrence.
- Obtaining another assessment.
- Follow-up.

Among the concerns parents express are fears about what will happen to the child in the next minute or the next day and what the child will look like in adulthood. You may be thinking, "Is the baby going to be here tomorrow?" but the parents may be pre-occupied with "What is he going to look like when he is twenty-one and retarded?"

Responding to parents' questions may pose a dilemma and result in a situation where no matter if you say too much or too little, if you are too positive or too negative you are in trouble. What do you do? Despite fears of impairing the bonding process or creating self-fulfilling prophecies, our guiding principle of professional responses has to be honesty. The information given reflects the recognition that this is the parents' child and that they have a right and need to know what to expect. However, we also avoid omniscient predictions and instead indicate that no one can precisely determine the future for any child born normal or otherwise. We should not go beyond our data nor should we fall short of it. We need to balance optimism and realism, the known with the unknown, and we should present our information in such a way as to foster constructive and thoughtful behavior on the parents' part. This means not saying things like, "He is going to ruin your family life. You should get rid of him." or, "Kids like this don't grow up to be anything, what are you wasting your time for?" You are well aware these are questions or statements that parents have heard. We can say instead, "You do not have to confront everything all at once about what your child is going to be like. Let's take it day by day. We're going to help you."

Parents are most worried that this condition might be the beginning of the end of their family life. They need to hear that this diagnosis does often represent a crisis in the lives of individuals and families; that having a lot of feelings of sadness, anger, or helplessness or the desire to get rid of the child does not mean they are mentally ill; and that it does not mean that things will not come into equilibrium again. They need to know that, with time and appropriate assistance, these reactions and stresses can usually be dealt with. You can also discuss costs and available benefits. Parents can be given specific guidance in relation to dealing with other children, with relatives, and with friends. They need to know that they are going to continue to need help, that it is not just all going to end.

A mother of a child with Down's syndrome wrote a book with

which you may be familiar, *The Gift of Martha*(4), in which she underscores the significance of presenting to parents the possibility that family members can grow and mature as an outcome of something that initially appears to be an unendurable tragedy. She writes:

> I will be the last person in the world to tell anyone that mental retardation is a happy circumstance. Yet if just one person had come to tell us that despite our sadness there was hope that this was not the end of the world but rather a challenge and unifying force, that this could bring out the best in each member of the family, how much more bearable our grief would have been.

That is, of course, stated in retrospect. Who knows if she would have been able to hear any of this or if people did not say that to her. But I think she is saying something important, that families can be helped, maybe even at an early stage, to see that perhaps growth can take place, as well as sadness, unhappiness, and problems, through the experience of having a handicapped child.

The issue of placement of the child out of the home is very complicated. Families have to know that achieving placement is a complex process, though they usually do not have to make this decision right away. Lifetime, permanent decisions can wait until they can work with their child, then gradually make the decisions out of the knowledge of the child, rather than out of a stereotype. Parents also need to know that the problems and feelings associated with the child rarely vanish when the placement is made, that the families often need help afterward, that having another baby immediately does not obliterate the experience or replace the child, and that they should take time for mourning and healing.

At this interview families may also ask why this happened and what the chances of its happening again are. We would prefer not to do genetic counseling at the informing interview, but often we cannot avoid saying some things. The main things that you want to say are, "Those are good questions. We know they are on your mind. We think they are deserving of a special interview, a separate time, a chance for us to get together all the information you want to have." Then schedule another appointment. Do not try to do genetic counseling in the middle of this interview that is dealing with much more immediate and pressing information. We also tell them that it would be best if they would postpone another pregnancy until the completion of genetic counseling but to contact the physician promptly if conception occurs in the interim before the appointment is made for genetic counseling.

We are very much in favor of offering parents the opportunity for a second opinion from a reputable source. We feel this is so important that we present this if the family itself does not ask, because then they know that it is all right to go elsewhere, that they are not going to lose our support, concern, and caring for them, that this is serious business and, therefore, they may want confirmation from another place.

We conclude the informing interview with the designation of a care coordinator and an outline of a plan of service for the immediate future. A plan is formed that includes well-child care, a habilitation, education, and development plan, and a psychosocial care plan. Available sources are identified and responsibilities for activating them are delineated. A structure for future contact with the family is defined so that there is a regular opportunity for the review of old issues and for the consideration of new ones.

This is the point where many plans fall down. We get to this point; everything seems to be done, and somehow parents go off into the night. Three years later they surface and they have had a horrible time. We believe, therefore, that the content of the informing interview should be summarized in a written report to the parents, including a plan for ongoing dialogue and contact. The report helps them to reflect on information and formulates a basis on which to continue working with professionals, whether the medical providers and other providers are the same or change. We also tell them, by sending a report, that they are part of the team for the care of their child. This may be a very different kind of feeling than they have ever had before in their relationships with professionals.

All of what has happened in the informing process is going to be reviewed and expanded periodically, because parents cannot and do not have to come to terms with everything all at once. They have and need their whole lives to do so. We need continuing opportunities for interaction between parents and professionals because what is being said needs to be integrated and because the developmental needs of all family members continually change(5). The early period between identification and the informing interview should set the stage for the provision of continuing supportive services to child and family that are vital for coping.

TRAINING HEALTH PROFESSIONALS ABOUT FAMILIES

Because this is not purely a medical problem, persons in the health care professions often feel inadequate to deal with the complex feelings and responses of the family to this devastating event. Such a birth demands from the physician good communication skills, sensitivity, and a sense of timing. The presentation of diagnosis with the first counseling session is a critical encounter because the long-term adjustment to the handicapped child begins at this time. The goal of the physician and the health care team (and I emphasize *team* although I think it will many times be done only by a physician) is to provide enough information and support to the family that they can begin to adjust rationally to the problems at hand. Of prime importance is the recognition by all involved of the great degree of psychological trauma experienced by the family and the need for the establishment of a foundation for the family's continuing emotional support. All of this raises the question of how pediatric faculty teach "competency blended with compassion." How do you train people to do all these wonderful things that we have said need to be done(6, 7)?

People who are concerned with the welfare of handicapped children and their families point out that the training, the awareness, the sensitivity, and the skills of pediatricians are often not adequate to meet the needs of these families. It is not surprising to note that following medical school, pediatric residency is generally directed to the care of hospitalized patients and, when there is time allowed, to ambulatory care. In a busy clinic or in an emergency room, efforts are directed toward the management of a single acute illness. This is the same sort of situation that exists in other programs such as nursing, occupational therapy, and physical therapy. The majority of pediatricians in training today will be expected to function as members of a team of professionals, jointly overseeing the health and developmental needs of children, particularly children under the age of five. They will function not only as consultant and counselor to individual children and their families but also as coordinator of effective delivery of services through a variety of community facilities. The pediatrician who deals with handicapped children will have an impact on what goes on in the care of these children not only in his own office but also in the community, by what he recommends and supports.

Thus we are looking at not only teaching the skills necessary for a health professional to function from the time that the baby is born in the delivery room(8) but also teaching the skills that go from delivery room to informing interview to counseling session, to follow-up, to follow-up, to follow-up, and to follow-up. We have to teach the health care professionals how to function as a part of a team of professionals, not a team composed solely of their own discipline but of other disciplines as well.

How do you conceptualize a teaching of competency and compassion? How do you teach a person to be a good clinician and to have interpersonal skills? Begin by teaching the staff to give adequate information. More important than what the family remembers is their perception of adequacy. The family needs to feel that they "got the whole story," or "got what we needed to know." But the amount of information delivered by physicians at the time of an informing interview is generally determined by how much the physician thinks the parents already suspect. If something is obvious because of congenital malformations, physicians are much more likely to give the right amount of information, because there is no hiding the obvious. The literature, though sparse in this area, confirms that fact. Physicians are much less likely to give full information in situations where the baby was born looking all right but where resuscitation was necessary and lengthy, or where the baby was worked on after it was shown briefly to the mother, then rushed to intensive care while the mother was taken up to her floor.

The amount of information given is also determined in part by the severity of the diagnosis. If it is clear that the child is going to need special kinds of treatment, facilities, care, or special schooling, the physician may give more information. He knows that the parents are going to eventually learn that a doctor has been less than frank with them if he does not give all the information at that time.

It is fascinating to look at the reasons people give for telling or not telling certain things. The amount of information delivered has been shown, for example, to be determined by the clinician's perception of parental level of adjustment. Parents perceived as coping well are told a lot more than others. This approach backfires, however, because many parents who received inadequate information report that the physician's vagueness made them much more anxious and upset. Those parents perceived as unable to handle the information found their stress heightened by the withholding of information.

We can talk to clinicians in training situations about reasons for presenting certain kinds of information, how much to give, what variables may influence decisions, and about the manner of presentation. But how can parental adjustment be assessed so that information can be delivered helpfully?

Repetition is important. A single informing interview is not enough. Information has to be repeated, and at every visit it is important to ask the parents for a restatement in order to assess parental understanding; otherwise it is possible to walk in on a fourth follow-up visit with some parents, assuming that they know what is wrong with their child and find that they do not. They may not have heard the first, second, and third time. So you should ask them to restate what they heard the time before. I would also recommend that you use a written statement, although it can in no way take the place of oral repetition and parental restatement.

The person who does the helping should have empathy, respect, and genuineness. Genuineness has been related in the psychological literature to self-disclosure(9). How do you present yourself as a genuine human being? That is something I think that we can teach. Empathy and sensitivity can be taught.

The clinician must have a positive attitude in characterizing the handicapped child. This is a prerequisite to adequate care that gives support to the family. Such attitudes can be developed.

The important points to remember are the need for information to be repeated and restated and the need for empathy and a positive, open attitude.

REFERENCES

1. Irvin, N. A., Kennell, J. H., & Klaus, M. H. Caring for parents of an infant with a congenital malformation. In M. H. Klaus & J. H. Kennell (Eds.), *Maternal-infant bonding: The impact of early separation or loss on family development.* St. Louis: Mosby, 1976, pp. 183–184.
2. Kennell, J. H., & Rolnick, A. R. Discussing problems in newborn babies with their parents. *Pediatrics,* 1960, *26,* 837.
3. Fox, A. M. *They get this training but they don't really know how you feel.* West Sussex, England: National Fund for Research into Crippling Diseases (Vicent House, Springfield Road), 1974, p. 30.
4. Canning, C. *The gift of Martha.* Boston: Children's Hospital Medical Center, 1975.
5. Turnbull, A. P., & Turnbull, H. R., III. *Parents speak out: A view from the other side of the two-way mirror.* New York: Merrill, 1978.
6. Richardson, H. B., Guralnick, M. J., & Tupper, D. B. Training pediatricians for effective involvement with handicapped pre-school children and their families. *Mental Retardation,* 1978, *16,* 3–7.
7. Kupst, M. J., Dresser, K., Schulman, J. L., & Paul, M. H. Evaluation of methods to improve communication in the physician-patient relationship. *American Journal of Orthopsychiatry,* 1975, *45,* 420–429.
8. Bocian, M., & Kaback, M. Crisis counseling: The newborn infant with a chromosomal abnormality. *Pediatric Clinics of North America,* 1978, *25,* 643–650.
9. Jourad, S. M. *The transparent self.* New York: Van Nostrand, 1971.

14

a care-by-parent unit

BILL S. CALDWELL

Bill S. Caldwell, PhD, is *Director of Psychology in the Department of Pediatrics, University of Texas Medical Branch in Galveston, Texas. He gives the history of and describes a special hospital unit where parents are responsible for providing most of the care and services. Responses to a questionnaire assessment of parent satisfaction are included.*

We spent approximately three years planning the Care-By-Parent Unit through meetings with hospital administrators, physicians, medical administrators, and insurance companies. We visited the two existing units(1, 2), one of which has gone out of existence. At the end we agreed on certain policies that would guide the unit, and these policies are still in existence. One, there would be no nursing personnel on the unit, none. Two, the unit would be open to all services that could qualify according to the admitting criteria so it would not be confined to orthopedics or to nephrology or to one of the other services, but it would be open to all services if the patients could qualify. Three, the parent or other designated caretaker would be responsible for the child twenty-four hours a day, and the parents could not delegate this authority to anyone else. Parents could not leave and say, "Mrs. Jones, will you take care of my child while I am gone?" This is not allowed. Parents are responsible for their child twenty-four hours a day. The fourth policy was that there would be a unit coordinator who would be the only hospital personnel on the unit, and who would function under written policies. The only person who could bend a policy would be the chair of our Care-By-Parent Committee or someone designated by that chair but no one else.

The unit operates like this: If a physician wishes to admit a child, he or she writes a protocol telling why the child should be admitted to this unit, listing the probable diagnosis and any unusual circumstances that might take place. Unusual circumstances might be that the child is subject to seizures or that the child is on some medication and there is a possibility there will be some unforeseen reaction to that medication. The protocol is submitted to the unit coordinator and, if it comes within the guidelines of the unit, the child is admitted. If there is a difference of opinion as to whether the child should be admitted or not, the unit coordinator calls the person who chairs the Care-By-Parent Committee to make the decision. Someone from the committee is always available as a backup to the unit coordinator.

There have been a few differences of opinion, though not too many. One day one of our physicians called and told the unit coordinator that he would like to admit a child. He submitted his protocol and she said, "I'm sorry, Doctor, I just don't think this meets our criteria." And he said, "Well, I have to get this child in the hospital. There are no other beds available. You have a bed available, and I know it." And she said, "Yes, we do, but it does not meet the criteria." So he called our chairman who happened to be a good friend, and he said, "I have a child I have to put in your unit." And she said, "Tell me about the child." So he talked and talked, and she said, "I'm not sure that this meets our criteria. By the way, is this an emergency?" And he said, "It certainly is." And she said, "Well, now I know it doesn't, because we have a policy that says that we will admit no emergencies." He laughed and took it good-naturedly and said, "Next time it won't be an emergency."

We have found it necessary to have rather strict policies and to stick with them. Otherwise the unit would stay filled up with children who were simply waiting to be transferred to somewhere else. It would become just a holding tank, and we did not want that. We will not allow that.

Once admitted to the unit, the child is under the care of the parent. The parent is in charge of carrying out the duties that the nurse ordinarily would carry out. The parents do not have the skill of a nurse, you know that, or the knowledge, but they are still responsible for carrying out the light housekeeping duties, such as changing the linens on the bed and keeping the place cleaned up. The housekeeping staff does the heavy cleaning work, but the parent takes care of the child.

Meals are served on the unit from the hospital kitchen. However, we do have a refrigerator and a microwave oven so that parents can prepare light snacks. We also have a washer and dryer on the unit. We do not have apartments; we could not afford that, so the family lives in one room. We have room for two parents and a child in each room. If both parents are not available we would have room for another person, but we would not use the extra space for a sibling. The mother or father is in charge of the hospitalized child, and we felt that having a sibling would take up their time. Since the siblings are not ill, they need something to do all day. We felt siblings would just create problems, so we drew our limit there.

The reason we do not have a nurse as the unit coordinator is that first, it is hard to get nurses and second, we are trying to reduce cost. We thought of what service we could dispense with without lowering the care of the patient to a critical level. Our patients are children who are not acutely ill and who would be taking the time of the nurse unnecessarily if they were on the children's unit. For example, a child waiting for certain types of surgery, a child with a chronic illness, a child who is there for educational purposes, a child with a cleft lip, or a newborn whose mother has to learn how to feed the baby might be on the unit.

For these particular types of patients we felt that the parents could provide the care. The way we arrived at this conclusion was very simple: the parents provided this care at home anyway. If they have a child who is, we will say, a child with diabetes, then either the child or the parent is already giving the injections, so this is not a new role for them.

QUESTION: What, then, is the reason to be a hospital patient?

CALDWELL: We see a lot of children with diabetes who have gone out of control, for example.

QUESTION: You have children with diabetes who have gone out of control in this unit.

CALDWELL: Oh, yes.

QUESTION: It must be different from ours; ours are very sick.

CALDWELL: If they are acutely ill they would not go in here. You know and I know that there is a variation of children out of control—if they are comatose, no. Suppose this child is getting out of control, reacting adversely to a dysfunctional family. We see a number of children like that. In this unit we can study the family and talk with them, since it is an educational as well as a care unit. A dietitian can come in and start working with the child and the family. Again, let me say that when we decided not to have nursing staff it was not easy to answer all the questions that nurses raised, although the particular nurse on our committee is in full agreement with that decision. We had to think of such things as emergencies. For emergencies we have a hot line phone; every parent knows where it is. It is connected directly to a nursing station so all they have to do is pick it up and start talking. It is a true hot line, and if it is a true emergency they will get an emergency response.

Incidentally, we have had no emergencies on this unit. This may sound strange but we are very careful about our selection of patients. The only incident we had that some people thought was an emergency was when a child had a seizure. The parent did not think it was an emergency because she dealt with seizures all the time.

The physician writes the purposes for the hospitalization in his protocol. If he needs a nutritionist or a dietitian to teach a mother how to feed her baby, he writes it in his orders and arrangements are made. I do not mean to say that no other hospital person ever comes around; I am simply saying they are not on duty there. We certainly use the services of other hospital personnel. An occupational therapist or physical therapist might come in; a psychologist like myself comes for the children with behavioral disorders. It is according to the need.

The coordinator of the unit, therefore, must have a wide understanding of the hospital and be acquainted with the resources, policies, and knowledge of how this particular hospital functions, including some of the pressures and the politics. The coordinator must have skill in working with various people.

The unit is under the direction of a committee composed of four physicians, a social worker, a pharmacist, a nurse—we did not forget them, see—two hospital administrators, and a psychologist.

The committee is charged with monitoring the costs of the day-to-day operation of the twelve rooms, formulating policy, interpreting the operation of the unit to both professionals and nonprofessionals, and acting as the liaison between that unit and everyone else.

Our physicians are well aware of the unit; they realize that they need to answer immediately when they get a call. They will not get a call unless it is a true emergency. Some of the problems we faced, however, were with our physicians. All physicians are accustomed to writing orders and having nurses carry them out or interpret them or supervise the carrying out of orders. Now, the parents carry out the orders. Quite strange. So we had to talk about that. We had to talk about such problems as prepping a child for surgery. Where do you do this? The first time this came up, the surgeon called down and wanted to know where his patient was. The unit coordinator answered, "Well, your patient's down here in the unit." He said something about the nurse, and she said, "We don't have nurses." "Who's going to do this?" the doctor asked, and the coordinator said, "I'm sure I don't know." He was a good surgeon and he said, "Hell, I'll do it myself." So the first thing we knew he was down there with transportation brought by himself, did the work himself, and out he went with the child. I am not saying all surgeons do this, but this showed that there is a way to handle these incidents. The surgeons and house staff have been very cooperative; they have adjusted to this nontraditional way of caring for children. It is quite different from picking up the phone and leaving an order and having everything done for you.

Once the unit was in operation we began to look at the cost. We studied a six-month period one year after the unit had started operation. In this six-month period there was an increase of 399 patient days in the unit over the previous six months. We use this as an indication of success; an increase of usage, for us, is an indicator of success. For this six-month period the average cost to the hospital per patient day was $132.23. On a comparative regular pediatric unit in the same six months the cost per patient day was $222.32. We considered a ninety dollar per patient per day reduction to be significant.

Next we polled physicians to see what they thought of the unit. Forty-seven of the fifty-seven physicians felt that their patients received as good medical care on this unit as on any other unit. Two felt that it was better. Thirty-six of the physicians said that they spent the same amount of time with the patient on the unit as they had on regular units. Fifteen physicians said it took more time, and four said it took less time than on regular units.

In comparison with a regular unit, the physicians thought that procedures were performed more conveniently thirty-four times and less conveniently twenty-three times. So despite the variation there, a preponderance of the physicians felt that a procedure could be performed more conveniently on the Care-By-Parent unit.

Of the fifty-seven physicians who admitted the sixty-nine children we studied, fifty-six of them said they would admit their patients again to the unit. We thought that was a good percentage.

Our house staff has been very fine. They come to sit and talk with their patients and the parents. Almost any time of the day you could go by there and see one of our house staff sitting there just talking.

We have a large lounge that has become a meeting place, where the parents come to talk, play cards, and exchange ideas and information. It is more like home, a pleasant place. No parent is going to sit and watch the child all the time. The children play in the hall or in the room. If the children need to be watched, the parent has to watch them, but most of the children are not that ill. They may be running around with an intravenous in their arm, but so what? They would be running around anyway.

In other parts of the hospital, although parents spend the night with their children, they are not involved in care to the extent that they are on this unit.

The impact on the child has been tremendous, the response has been tremendous, and I do not think there is any question but that it is preferable to the way children are usually hospitalized. You cannot bring all of the home into the hospital, there is no way to do that, but this unit brings part of the home into the hospital and that is important to the child.

QUESTION: If you have an infant admitted for failure-to-thrive and you have the parent there doing all the care, who is there observing what is going on between the parent and the child?

CALDWELL: This is one of the reasons for developing this unit, to give us a chance to observe. The social worker, the psychologist, or someone working with them, maybe one of my Fellows in psychology, maybe one of our social work graduate students would go there.

COMMENT: You see, I am used to the nurse being the one.

CALDWELL: I know you are. We simply work it out so that the person who is working with that patient finds the time to observe. As you have noticed, some of the people whom we have admitted here are children with behavior problems, whether they are listed this way or not. We do our own observation of them.

QUESTIONNAIRE RESULTS

We developed a questionnaire, which 156 parents completed, to assess the attitudes of parents who have stayed on the unit. Here are some of the results: To the question, "Did your doctor tell you why your child was being admitted?", 139 parents said yes.

The next question we asked was, "Did you get information about the unit itself?" Over half of the parents responding did not get complete information about the unit. We had asked the physicians to describe the unit, but not all of them did. Sometimes parents told their doctors that they understood when they did not.

We asked, "Did you get enough information about the unit when your child entered?" Information is given by both the physician and the unit coordinator before the family actually settles in on the unit. Four parents said they got little information; that is where we slipped up, and we used these questionnaires to self-correct as we went along. Self-correction is one of the reasons for administering these questionnaires, and the parents were quite willing to fill them out. We asked questions about their satisfaction with the unit, about the parents' feelings about working with their child, about their being "Comfortable" or "Uncomfortable" and "Confident" or "Not Confident." Ten of the parents said they were not confident about doing these things for their child, but most of them felt comfortable and confident.

We asked, "Did you feel confined with twenty-four-hour-a-day care?" Six said they certainly felt confined, and I think I would agree with them that it is confining, but most of them did not feel confined. I think this shows that, although they were confined, they felt good about being there. I think we are getting a halo effect here.

We asked, "Did you feel better about doing these things at the beginning of your child's stay or at the end?" The median answer there was, "I felt good at the beginning and at the end, both. It made no difference; I did not change my feeling. I was so glad to be here with my child." Other people felt better at the beginning; by the time they had been there four or five days with their child, twenty-four hours a day, they were ready to get out. Most of the children were with us from three to six days. Getting bored was the chief complaint we have had from the parents.

The next was a global question, "Were you satisfied?" Most of them were satisfied, even those who said that they felt confined or did not feel confident. Most of them were very positive in their responses to the unit. They were very happy with it. We got very few dislikes. What they really liked though was that it was a place where they could stay with their child. Cost was not as important as we thought it might have been; ninety-seven out of these 156 parents, however, did say that it was important.

"What did you dislike?" Four of them wanted nurses. One person said that this was too much responsibility; this parent was not happy with our unit and told us that she was not happy from the time she entered until the time she left. She brought her child to the hospital to be taken care of; she did not want the responsibility; she did not want the problems; she wanted somebody else to take care of her child. But this was the great exception.

We asked, "If your child is taking medicines, did someone talk to you about the medicine?" Seven said "no," the rest "yes."

We also used a questionnaire with our children and adolescents. Obviously a child has to be able to read to answer this, so we did not get responses from nonreaders. There were very few dislikes by the children. They were happy to have their parents stay. Dislikes mentioned were the food, the bed not being comfortable, and sharing a bathroom.

Now, what did they like? "Could be with mommy," was a response we received over and over. "I could take a bath when I wanted to," "I got to wear my own clothes; it wasn't like a hospital," and so forth. They were responding to the fact that this was more like home than it was like a hospital. Most of the children had been hospitalized in traditional units before.

Privacy was mentioned by many children. The quietness was appreciated by many children. The lack of rush and bustle that we sometimes find in hospitals is absent here, and children respond positively to that.

I think most of you understand the problems with using questionnaires. You get halo effects; you get all sorts of effects that you wish you did not get. But we did not have the personnel to carry out private interviews with these parents. We would have preferred that. Also, these are self-completion questionnaires. That is why I say they have their drawbacks.

Ninety-nine of these 156 patients had been hospitalized before. Of the twelve parents who said they would have preferred a regular pediatric ward or room, most of them gave the explanation, "My child was acutely ill," or "seriously ill" or "really ill," and that is why they gave that preference. Of those who went through the hospitalization on the unit, 143 said they preferred the unit. Again, most of them had been on other units.

Someone asked what else the parents do. They take vital signs. Not all of them take blood pressure because sometimes blood pressures were done by people who are in training here. But all of the parents were trained to do these various procedures, which they might do at home, with the exception of watching an IV at home.

QUESTION: But how could there be an IV? I mean, who is the one starting that—the doctor is going to stay there for eight hours to run one monitor?

CALDWELL: No, he does not stay there; the parents are the ones who are going to watch the IV.

QUESTION: Who changes the bottles?

CALDWELL: No, the parents will not do that. They will watch the bottle, however.

QUESTION: What happens if an IV infiltrates? What do they do?

CALDWELL: They would pick up the hot-line phone. What I am saying is that we have not had any emergencies on that unit.

QUESTION: So an IV infiltrating would be an emergency? And all the IVs have run well?

CALDWELL: Again, folks, you are asking questions in terms of nursing care. If you will think in terms of a sick child at home, what does a parent do with a sick child at home? What happens if you have a child on medication? You say, "You must give this medication every four hours." Parents get up and they give the medication. In addition to this, they take their child to occupational therapy or physical therapy or to the lab, collect stool specimens, and on and on. But these are some of the more common things that the parents were doing. The hospital and the physician still have the responsibility, we know this.

QUESTION: Why did you decide not to have a nurse in attendance.

CALDWELL: We were trying to balance nursing care with cost, and we opted to go with lower cost. In addition, there is a nursing shortage as you all know. I would be foolish to say that a nurse could not have helped. I would also be foolish to believe, however, that nursing care is essential on this unit. We have now run the unit for almost two years and, to be very honest, we have not really felt that we have lost a great deal by not having nurses.

We have no plans right now to add a nurse. It is different from a unit with acutely ill patients.

We are not using volunteers right now. Few of the children have complained about having nothing to do; the parents have, but not the children. The children are meeting new people, getting acquainted, talking, watching TV, playing games with toys, and roaming around the hospital if they are old enough.

We have some nursing students who are learning to work with children, and they play with them some. We do not have a director of activities. Remember, it is like being in the home. You would not think of organizing a family because you have different age children. Here the older children take care of the younger children and show them how to do things, teach them. It becomes like a family.

REFERENCES

1. Green, M., & Green, J. G. The parent care pavilion. *Children Today,* Sep–Oct 1977, *6,* 5–9.
2. James, V. L., & Wheeler, W. E. The care by parent unit. *Pediatrics,* 1969, *43,* 488–494.

unit D

MUTUAL-SUPPORT
PARENT GROUPS

15

a staff-directed group for parents of neurologically impaired children

BLANCHE B. VALANCY

Blanche B. Valancy, ACSW, is a Social Worker at Cleveland Metropolitan General Hospital in Ohio. She describes the formation, operation and content of groups designed to enable parents to understand and cope with their children's disabilities.

As we tried to assist parents through their child's hospitalization and subsequent care, we were aware of their many difficulties. Parents were doubtful of their ability to carry out medical regimens. They expressed feelings of isolation, loneliness, and unresolved guilt over the birth of a handicapped child. Parents who reported increased marital and family problems attributed them to the presence of the chronically ill child in the family and to the need to give extra time and special attention to that child over and above the siblings. Parents also expressed anger with the child, anxiety about the future, depression, resentment, or unresolved guilt and grief.

It soon became clear that the professionals were not able to give the needed support, understanding, and specific practical suggestions that grow only out of having a similar life experience. One mother told me that she thought there needed to be a group for parents whose children had neurological problems. If she could only attend such a group, she said, she might not feel so alone and overwhelmed by her child's problems. If her husband could only attend such a group, perhaps he would begin to recognize and even admit that their child had a problem.

A graduate student who was doing her field work in child neurology at our hospital helped us form just such a group. A year later I formed a second group along with a nurse who had considerable experience with disabled children.

These short-term parent groups filled some of the cognitive needs of parents, in such areas as caretaking skills, awareness of community resources, understanding of the health care system, and the roles and limitations of health professionals. The groups also satisfied some of the parents' affective needs in the areas of communication skills, feelings about parental roles, feelings of sorrow, isolation, depression, guilt, and anxiety.

We decided that co-leadership of the group was essential. Each leader could support the other. Two leaders could be more aware of the events occurring in the group and could work together to keep the discussion on the track better than one group leader could. It also seemed that dividing the power implicit in the role of leader would prevent our being given too much individual power and allow us to be group members ourselves.

THE GROUP MODEL

This small, discussion-educational group, formed to provide mutual assistance to its members who share a stressful life situation has been described as a "situation/transition group(1)." There are five essential features that define the composition of these groups.

First, these groups are primarily oriented toward helping members cope more effectively with a shared external event, for example, a medical problem, job, or stage of life such as widowhood or the birth of a first child. They are not oriented toward insight, change, or social action, as would be a therapy group. Second, they involve five to twelve members and meet from one to two hours per week over a period of four to fifteen weeks. Thus they have a limited membership and are time-limited groups. Third, these groups are moderated by a trained leader. In this way, they differ from self-help groups. Leaders of situation/transition groups tend to act more as peers, consultants, expediters, or facilitators, rather than as directive leaders such as you might find in a therapy group. Fourth, situation/transition groups offer social support, factual information about the shared life stress, and the opportunity for emotional interaction with other members. Fifth, these groups do not encourage or require members to espouse a particular moral or behavioral value system as do groups that are concerned with growth or change.

This type of group fills a very important function in primary prevention of emotional disturbances. By providing a social resource to satisfy the member's needs for support, self-esteem, knowledge, group identification, and social interaction, the group helps to equip its members to withstand current and future stresses and crises.

The group leader must understand this distinction between therapy and prevention in order to determine the focus of group discussion, to avoid inappropriate probing, and to prevent the more powerful group members from taking control of the group and having their needs met at the expense of the other members.

FORMING THE GROUP

We then developed the criteria for membership and the methods for recruitment. The situation/transition group model calls for a shared life stress, so we decided that the ages and the medical problems of the children should be similar. We recruited parents, therefore, of preschool children who had diagnoses of brain damage. We urged parents who were living together as couples to attend as couples, hoping thereby to discuss the marital stresses implicit in the situation.

Membership in the group was closed; once meetings had started, we did not add any new members. We felt this would keep intragroup commitment high. By not bringing in "strangers" more group spirit would develop.

In the situation/transition model, group life is time-limited, so parents were informed of the projected termination date during our pregroup interviews and the termination date was repeated at each meeting. We felt this time-limitation would also keep the interest and involvement high because the members would know that they only had a limited time to discuss what they felt was important. Pregroup interviews were held with all potential members to give us an opportunity to assess the appropriateness of group membership for the parents in terms of the similarity of the children, as well as allowing us to screen out any parents who seemed to exhibit pathological reactions to their children's handicaps or serious social, emotional, or marital problems. We felt that members who were unstable would not best be served by a group, would be upsetting to the other members, and would disrupt the group process.

During the pregroup interviews we also explained our ideas about the purpose of the group and solicited the parents' ideas, thoughts, and concerns, which we noted and brought up for discussion during group meetings. Out of those concerns we developed a list of goals and means by which we, as leaders, intended to approach the goals.

GOALS OF THE GROUPS

Three of the goals were to meet the cognitive needs of the parents or the objective learning needs, and three other goals were to meet affective or subjective or emotional support needs of the parents.

The first cognitive goal was improvement of their caretaking skills, which we approached through education, recruiting outside experts to speak to the group on such areas as speech pathology, psychology, and physical therapy. We discussed caretaking roles and parent satisfaction with their roles. We encouraged the attendance of both parents to try to promote some solidarity between them, and we discussed problems in the parent-child relationship such as methods of discipline and toilet training.

Our second cognitive goal was to increase the parents' awareness of community resources, which we did by simply discussing available resources at the hospital and through our community agencies. Our third cognitive goal was to increase the members' understanding of health professionals and their roles and limitations. To do this, we conducted discussions aimed at further delineating the roles of the different people they would meet in the hospital. As a spinoff of this we hoped to increase the understanding that the health professionals themselves, at least the ones who spoke with the group, had of the parents. I do not know of any way to assess that understanding; I wish I did because I am hoping that the professionals heard some of what the parents had to say about how they would like us, as professionals, to be behaving toward them.

The first of the affective goals was to reduce parental feelings of isolation and stigma. Just getting together a group of people whose problems were similar was helpful. Now parents could say, "I know somebody else in my situation." We also provided an atmosphere in which the discussion of either positive or negative feelings was acceptable.

Our second affective goal was to increase the parental comfort with, and satisfaction derived from, the neurologically impaired child. When the group met, the parents had time away from the children. In some cases, especially the mothers, this was the only time all month that they left the child in the care of others, giving them increased comfort through distance. Finding out that someone else could take care of the child, yet the relationship would still be there when the family returned home, was reassuring. We hoped also to increase parental comfort by providing them with an opportunity to express their feelings about their children, by supporting the legitimacy of those feelings, and by supporting their recognition of their useful defenses.

Our third affective goal was the improvement of communication skills between both parents, between the parents and the child, between the parents and the siblings of the child, between parents and their friends and relatives, and between parents and strangers. We approached this goal through modeling, by using good communication skills, and by discussion of actual situations that the parents had experienced.

OUTCOME OF THE GROUPS

We met twice a month for seven meetings (the first group) and eight meetings (the second group). The parents spoke of problems at the time of diagnosis and hospitalization, confusion about which staff did what task, frustrations and fears for their children's future, feelings about not being able to do enough to make up to the child for his disability, the need to function as a couple, and handling the reactions and comments of others in the family, and strangers who ask questions.

At the last meeting of each group we asked the members to evaluate the group experience and to compare their thoughts and feelings at the end with their thoughts and feelings on the first night. Parents generally agreed that they had moved from feeling very nervous, scared, and skeptical to being much more comfortable and relaxed. Parents said they enjoyed the group meetings and looked forward to them as a good opportunity to get out of the house and do something constructive. The parents stated that they had learned from each other and that they felt less alone than they had before. The group was valuable, they said, because they had obtained factual information and had a forum for expressing their thoughts and feelings.

As leaders, we were impressed with how well and quickly the group formed, integrated, and got down to business. There was almost none of the storming or conflict period that we had expected there would be at the beginning of the life of a group.

There might be three possible reasons for this early cohesiveness and lack of tension. First, the pregroup selection and orientation assured us a group of well-motivated and appropriate members. All the parents had understood from the pregroup interviews what the goals of the group were, and they knew that their ideas and their problems were the focus of the meetings. Secondly, we spent a great deal of time getting organized for each meeting, cutting out a lot of floundering time that might have occurred otherwise. A third reason for the cohesiveness came about because we sent letters summarizing each meeting and stating our plans for the next one. We put these letters together from the audio tapes of the meetings. It took a lot of time; a two-hour meeting demanded two hours or more of listening to the tape, taking notes, and figuring out what happened. The letters summarized the process of the meeting and demonstrated our acceptance of the thoughts and feelings that had been expressed by making them important enough to put them down on paper. There is something about seeing on paper what you said and did that gives legitimacy to it.

I believe the experience of our two groups of parents of neurologically impaired children demonstrates the efficacy of the situation/transition group model for working with parents in a medical setting. These parents were able to share knowledge, experience and learning situations with one another.

It is natural to be uneasy at the thought of meeting with clients in a group; however, a group that is carefully composed, with attention to planning and to organization all through the group's life, can be a rewarding experience for the leader as well as for the members. It can also be a valuable service the medical institution can offer its consumers.

In order to organize our thinking in terms of the goals, functions, and even the composition of the group, we reviewed some reading material in the areas of psychological impact on families, specific neurological information, and group work theory. A summary of this writing may be of help at this point.

DISCUSSION OF LITERATURE

Most writers concerned with the subject of disabled children and their families have pointed out the tragedy of the birth of a defective infant. In a landmark article called "Mourning and the Birth of a Defective Child," Solnit and Stark(2) based their theoretical approach on the psychoanalytic explanation of the process of mourning. A severe blow is dealt to the parents' normal narcissism because the discrepancy between the wish for a perfect child and the arrival of a damaged child is too great to be tolerated. The trauma is greater for the mother in most cases, they say, because of the normal loosening up of ego defenses and the more direct access to unconscious wishes and fears that is inherent normally in any pregnancy. The birth of the impaired child represents a sudden loss, or "death," of the perfect infant and its replacement by a feared, threatening, and possibly anger-provoking child. The lost baby must be mourned because a valued love object has been lost and grief is the normal reaction. But there is no time to work through the loss of the desired child before it is necessary for the parent to love the damaged child. Parents' normal grief and anger about what has happened is complicated by the fact that the baby they hoped for is not really dead, but rather a disabled living child who remains as a constant reminder of their loss. And they must learn to accept and nurture this child.

Olshansky(3) conceptualized the normal adjustment to the birth of a defective child as "chronic sorrow." He emphasizes the importance of recognizing the state of chronic grief as a natural, rather than a neurotic, response to the tragic reality if someone is to help the parents. Some parents exhibit pathological adjustments when they are not able to integrate the handicapped child into their reality. These can be placed on a continuum. At one end are parents whose extreme guilt feelings lead them to dedicate their entire existence to the care of the handicapped child to the exclusion of everyone else in the family and all other outside activities. At the other extreme is the parent who is so intolerant of the child that he or she gives in to the impulse to deny any relationship with the child. This is where we sometimes see parents, usually fathers, deserting families a year or so after a disabled child is born or the handicap is diagnosed. Both of these reactions indicate that an intolerable, narcissistic injury has been suffered, and the reactions probably reflect the parent's impaired self-image or coping ability before the birth of the baby. The birth of a defective child creates a crisis in normal development for the parents as individuals, for the marital pair, and for the family as a unit.

Miller(4) suggests five stages of parental adjustment. In stage one the parents are in shock and disintegration. In stage two, parents may deny anything is wrong. So much energy is needed to deal with their overwhelming emotions that little energy is left for coping with the environment. The third stage, sadness and anger, is the beginning of chronic sorrow. Parents waver between denial and acceptance and look for someone to blame. They may talk more about themselves than about the child and express much self-pity. In stage four, adaptation and adjustment, parents are becoming more realistic in their view of the problem and beginning to be able to plan. In stage five, reorganization and reintegration, parents' functioning is becoming more effective and more realistic. They are able to assign the handicapped child a place in the family. This stage is a goal in adjustment but occurs not very often in reality.

The literature also discusses some principles of informing and counseling parents of neurologically-impaired children. Solnit and Stark(2), in particular, point out the need for constant clarification of the reality of the child's condition as the parents are able to verbalize their questions and fears. This helps to strengthen their reality-testing abilities and to decrease distortions. They also point to the need for support and continuing clarification over a period of time. Our experience with the groups described here confirms these needs and supports the efforts of parents to cope more effectively.

REFERENCES

1. Schwartz, M. D. Situation/transition groups: A conceptualization and review. *American Journal of Orthopsychiatry,* 1975, *45,* 744–755.
2. Solnit, A. J., & Stark, M. H. Mourning and the birth of a defective child, *Psychoanalytic Study of the Child,* 1961, *16,* 523–537.
3. Olshansky, S. Chronic sorrow: A response to having a mentally defective child. *Social Casework,* 1962, *43,* 190–193.
4. Miller, L. Toward a greater understanding of the parents of the mentally retarded child. *Journal of Pediatrics,* 1968, *73,* 699–705.

16

a staff-directed
outpatient group
for parents
of children
with arthritis

IRA KURLAND

Ira Kurland, MSW, was a Clinical Social Worker for the Rheumatology Division and the Rehabilitation Center at Childrens Hospital, Los Angeles, California. He describes the process and content of group work with parents of children who have juvenile rheumatoid arthritis.

There are 250 patients with juvenile rheumatoid arthritis (JRA) who are actively followed at Childrens Hospital of Los Angeles, a center that receives referrals from all over the country and, on occasion, from outside the country.

The parents' group grew out of experience with other open-ended groups that I had established at the Rehabilitation Center for all hospitalized inpatients. Those groups pointed to the need for a therapeutic group for the JRA outpatient families.

The group met eight times from March through May, with new members joining anytime. The group met evenings to accommodate working mothers and fathers who often traveled from long distances.

All the parents were screened by this worker. The patients and their siblings stayed in the Rehabilitation Center while the group met, a very important service since baby-sitting was a problem. The group was co-led by a social work intern who also recorded the sessions.

Three people had previous group therapy experience which, I believe, made a difference in promoting conversation. At the beginning of the first group all of the parents told each other a little about themselves, their child, the illness, and the kinds of treatments their child was undergoing. This was an anxiety-provoking experience for all of them and there was a lot of hesitancy and voices cracking. One father cried and could not easily regain composure of himself. He did, however, receive immediate and considerable emotional support and never failed to attend a group after that. This was especially important because this father did not live with his child who had JRA and had feelings he wanted to express in the group.

All the parents became involved with the group, sharing problems and concerns and helping others to solve problems. The universality of these parents' experience allowed them to relate to each other quickly. They seemed not to need a long period of testing.

All of the families related horror stories about the diagnostic process. JRA is not an easy diagnosis to make. To give two examples: one young mother was initially assured that her three-year-old was having emotional problems because he refused to walk and cried a lot. In another case a two-year-old girl with an unusual presentation of symptoms was referred to an orthopedist who told the parents that they were abusing their child and that was the reason for all of her symptoms.

THERAPEUTIC ISSUES

When parents discussed a problem, a blurring of roles could sometimes be sensed. Occasionally it was difficult to determine which was the parent's problem and which was the child's. All of the parents expressed guilt in different ways and about many different aspects of the illness, for example, about behavior management and general parenting techniques. On occasion the guilt was so overwhelming that parents had trouble adjusting to the diagnosis even when the child was doing well medically or adjusting well psychologically.

Parents talked about feeling like ogres who were stuffing pills down their kids' throats. They also worried about the side effects of medications that could occur at present or in the future. Some medications for arthritis may have long-term effects, so their concern may have been well-founded.

Managing physical therapy with the child produced guilt feelings in parents who reported that when the children hurt, it seemed cruel to make them do something that hurt even more. In addition, because these children must take long bus rides to and from special schools and do their homework and exercises, they become exhausted. Parents talked about their distress over the fact that this left no time for the rewarding part of parenting. They wanted some time for that, but when they took time out for fun they felt guilty about neglecting the physical therapy. And when they put their own needs before the children's needs, they felt guilt about that as well. All parents talked about the fact that they felt particularly guilty, that there must be something they were doing wrong when their children were not doing well medically, were losing weight, and generally looked sick.

Single parents or divorced mothers talked about the fact that ex-spouses or ex-partners would say, "There must be something you are doing wrong," so that whatever guilt they felt on their own was heightened. We talked about ways of handling this, for example, directing the anger at the ex-spouse. Parents also talked about the fact that when they engaged in normal physical activities like hiking or walking, they felt badly because they knew that either their children could not do it or could do it only with tremendous pain. They felt guilty when their children said to them "You're lucky, you look normal. Look at me."

The overriding feeling expressed about guilt was that if they have a child who is sick then there must be something wrong with them. Several parents in the group said that they felt that there must be something that they had done wrong at some point along the way and that the sins of the parents were being visited on the children.

The children's condition had a strong effect on family relationships, with marital problems mentioned often. In one group there were two divorces directly attributed to the extra stress of managing with a child with JRA. In addition there were other marital conflicts over such questions as how much time should go to the sick child and which parent should do what. Favoritism toward the child who was sick was felt to be inevitable. On the other hand there were also several parents who expressed anger and frustration with the sick child. There was a good deal of sibling rivalry between the well child and the sick child.

Parents reported that their feelings of helplessness regarding the physical aspects of JRA were hard on them. JRA has its ups and downs, its relapses and remissions, and there is very little that the parent can do at some times. Until then, they had been looked on as problem-solvers by their children, they had felt omnipotent and now they were helpless. Emotionally they were not helpless, however, and they had many ways of helping the children to deal with the pain, by staying with them and by encouraging them to achieve in other areas. But in terms of the physical aspect of illness, they continued to feel very helpless.

The majority of the parents felt that there was an emotional element in either the cause or the relapses of the illness. They related it to changes in the family situation such as deaths, divorces, and other emotional turmoil within the family. This idea is not entirely accepted by the medical profession, but I want to mention it as something that the families often believed.

The fear of death was an issue that was dealt with from the third through the last session. Several JRA patients told their parents that they would rather be dead than in constant pain and chronically handicapped. Some parents handled this by telling their children how important they were to them. Other parents stayed with their children through the bad parts and let them know they could count on their parents no matter what. Some parents accented the good things, pointing out how much worse it could be and how the patients could more aggressively fight their illness. There was an attempt made to help the child separate himself from the illness; he is not juvenile rheumatoid arthritis, he is Johnny or Joe. Parents encouraged the anger, accepted the depression and frustration, and attempted to convey the feeling that no matter how bad it is now, things will get better. They also tried to help the children displace some of their anger either onto the parents or onto something to get them away from the depression.

One parent reported that when her child, who had severe systemic JRA, ran high fevers, "He had the smell of death." She remembered that her brother smelled that way just before he died. When this happened, she needed to get away, to go out and take a walk or to pray, but to get away for only a few minutes. Then she could come back and be a comfort and support to him. The feeling that he might die, which was reality-based, overwhelmed her.

The parents worried about what would happen to their children when they themselves died. Most of the parents felt that no one could help their children as well as they could. Several of them talked about the fact that they needed to keep themselves healthy. Others, however, invested a tremendous amount of their time and energy in the children and ignored that issue. The divorced parents felt more burdened by this. They did not have the family- or friend-support systems that the two-parent families seemed to have, and therefore they felt that if they were not there that the children would not be taken care of. Some families talked about moving here from far-flung areas and having trouble meeting new people. Two families had relocated to Southern California for treatment at Childrens Hospital, one from Tennessee and another from Israel. Others, however, said that they recognized that they were overly involved with their children, getting them to and from school and clinic appointments, getting their medications to them on time, helping them with their exercises and that they had purposely ignored their own socialization. The single-parent families felt more burdened by this, saying that they did not even have a spouse as one other adult for them to socialize with. They tended to ignore their own needs at work, school, or socialization. However, one single mother who said she would never be able to work because her child was a twenty-four hour, seven-day-a-week job was working and happier by session seven and she continues to work.

Parents of a child with this kind of illness experience many losses. The biggest loss is not having a basically healthy, normal child. No matter how well the child did after the diagnosis was made, even if the child was in total remission for long periods of time, these parents were never able to see the child as normal and healthy again. Denial was not something that we saw at all, at least not in this group population, and noncompliance was also not seen. I do think that there was some conscious suppression of fear, which allowed the children and the parents to engage in a more normal kind of functioning.

Parents and children needed outlets for physical expression. These children were limited in their ability to express themselves. They did not have sports or running or all of the other normal active outlets that most children have. Several of them had found negative forms of physical expression that were very difficult for the parents to deal with. Two of the girls kicked their fathers regularly, and one of the children threw food around. In discussing this all of the parents agreed that there was a need for physical expression by everyone, children and adults. Some ways of working this out were arranged. Those children who were able to manage bike riding and swimming lessons found these activities to be physically and psychologically therapeutic. Handicapped Scouting was useful for these physically disabled children who could not otherwise engage in scouting activities.

OUTCOMES OF THE GROUP

The parents evaluated the first eight sessions. They felt that there was a decided change in the clinic atmosphere, a warm, better feeling. They talked about the fact that the clinic was no longer such a bad place to go to, an activity to do alone with their sick child; instead there now tended to be clusters of families. There was the sense of an extended family where other members of the group tended to become honorary aunts and uncles. The concept of shared problems was seen as important in this group, but they talked about something more than that. They talked about the fact that at three o'clock in the morning, for example, if a child was crying out in pain and the parents had exhausted their repertoire of comforts, had already done everything that they could do for that child, when their best friends and family would not know how to help them, they could call other members of the group who could help them or could at least understand what they were going through at that point. The suggestion was made within the group for the development of a telephone hot line. Although this was optional and members had to decide whether or not they wanted to be available seven days a week, twenty-four hours a day, all of them did agree to it. It has been used since then.

Parents also learned varied coping methods. They talked about the fact that although they all had similar problems, they coped in different ways. Initially they felt that this difference was due just to individual differences. Later, they began to try different coping mechanisms that had been used by other parents and found them very helpful. There was a request that the group continue and that other families be invited to join. That request was met and we have been meeting twice a month since then, so the group is now a year-and-a-half old.

Parents talked about changes in their children. They felt that since they had been going to group that their children were better adjusted to the illness. One mother said that she thought there was a positive ripple effect from her going to group and suggested that the children should have a group also. (Just recently we did, in fact, have such a group. It was time-limited and has been completed successfully.)

Parents often reported that the group experience was the first opportunity they had where their needs were addressed. The members encouraged each other to take some time without the children, to go to school and work, to give their own feelings equal weight with those of their children. One parent reported that when she felt like crying she had always run into another room and hid from her child. She never felt she had the right to cry until the group leader helped her express her own feelings. When she finally did, her child said, "How did you control yourself so long? I was worried about you."

During the group sessions we talked about how the problems that these children had were not so very different from the problems that normal or healthy children had. As that came out in the group, the parents said that they felt that the problems were more manageable and that normal parenting activities could work for them.

Parents said they felt accepted in the group and could say things within the group that they had never talked about or dared to talk about before. This was carried over to home and often spouses would talk about the group for days afterward.

The group seemed to be both a beginning and a catalyst for opening communications within the family.

17

a parent-directed cardiology group

LINDA WILLIAMS AND RICHARD WITTNER

Linda Williams, BA, Parent Consultant for the American Heart Association, Long Beach, California, also chairs Parents With Hearts, an educational and mutual-support parent group in California. She describes the organization, its function, and its impact in helping families of children with heart problems.

Richard Wittner, MD, FACC, FAAP, is Director of Pediatric Cardiology at Earl and Loraine Miller Children's Hospital Medical Center in Long Beach, California. As the medical consultant to the organization, he describes the work of Parents With Hearts from a physician's viewpoint.

Parents With Hearts is an organization in Southern California for families who have children with congenital heart defects. We are a parent group, run by parents, with advice from the medical profession.

When our own child was born with a heart defect, we found three other families in the same situation and decided to form a group for mutual support. We approached feature writers of major newspapers in the area and told them what we were trying to do and how a support group could benefit other parents. Four newspapers ran half-page stories and the response was very good. Parents did want to learn more about their child's medical problem.

The Long Beach Heart Association agreed to help us with postage and flyers. We gave postcards with basic information about the group and a phone number to physicians who agreed to mail the cards to families they thought might be interested. Radio stations were also receptive; we taped interviews and spot announcements, and we were interviewed. We placed posters in the public libraries and listed our activities in their directories of community service organizations.

More families responded. Most of them came from Children's Hospital in Long Beach, others from ten area hospitals. The families had children from newborns to teenagers. Some children had defects that were corrected at an early age but the family was still in the group. Some children had had palliative surgery and were awaiting correction. Some defects were not correctable. Five families had lost their children but remained in the organization to be available for others in similar situations.

We offer two types of programs, a monthly rap session and an evening educational program. Children are frequently brought to the rap sessions. It helps parents to see another child who has the same condition and who has lived through heart surgery. It is reassuring to know that it is possible. Grandparents, friends, and neighbors are encouraged to attend the educational sessions as well. Professionals speak on topics such as "Procedures in the Operating Room," or "Physical and Emotional Development of a Child with Congenital Heart Defect." We have tours of the catheterization laboratory where the equipment is explained. We have also organized a library so that families can borrow books, articles, or tapes of selected programs.

The parents have grown in their ability to understand. Many comment that they can understand better at a parent program than they can in the doctor's office where their stress is greater.

To reach new families we now receive a copy of the surgery

schedule from the hospital. We then call the family and offer to send a parent to visit who has been through this and who handled the postoperative period well. This parent usually meets with the family again on the day of surgery.

We also have family fun activities such as a summer family picnic and a holiday party in December to help the siblings feel a part of the group.

A PHYSICIAN'S VIEWPOINT

From the group's beginning we have stressed understanding the problem and living with it. This is in contrast to other groups that emphasize the dying child. Since the prognosis has become more optimistic for children with congenital heart disease over the last forty years, we can today anticipate an almost normal life expectancy. So the interrelationship of the child with the parents, siblings, other relatives, and peers becomes more important.

There are unfortunately many children with congenital heart disease who are still treated as defective children with restrictions on schooling, physical education, and participation in activities. This is one aspect Parents With Hearts has looked at in order to improve the quality of life for these children and their families.

Parents With Hearts has helped physicians who deal with the medical and scientific aspects of child's problem. The group impresses on everyone around the child the importance of helping each child feel more like his peers than different from them.

The group gives parents an understanding of the child's problems. It gives information about normal heart murmurs, for instance, and the various problems that affect the child's heart and how the child's body deals with these particular problems.

I have heard of the impact of the group on the child from various stories. For example, one child was growing more withdrawn as she was upset about her scar until she saw another child at the meeting who also had a scar on her chest, then it was difficult to get her to put her shirt on again.

To be able to talk to a parent about the problem, using medical terminology, and for them to be able to use terminology like *palliative surgery* or *noncorrectable* or other scientific terms related to the child's defect, makes the whole situation much easier on the physician. The group has also helped me deal with children and parents on a day-to-day basis as well as in those very critical periods when the child is in the hospital for heart catheterization or surgery.

We have a very strong program at the hospital in our Child Life Program. Children who come in for cardiac catheterization and for surgery are oriented as to what they can expect, through puppet therapy and through photographs. It is difficult to know what part the parent group plays and what part our Child Life Program plays, but I think both are an integral part of dealing with the child who has a chronic problem. The child is very likely not going to have problems or symptoms on a day-to-day basis, so it behooves everyone working with the child to be very positive about rearing the child.

Today we can offer palliative or corrective surgery to ninety percent of youngsters with congenital heart problems. We are no longer looking at problems that occur in a year or two or three. We are looking instead at the problems that can be expected when they reach the teen years and beyond.

Many of the teens ask questions of the parents and of the physician. They want to know what can be expected when they are twenty-five and older. We talk about insurability and employability and marriage and pregnancy, not about death. Death as a result of congenital heart disease is behind us to a great extent and, we hope, will be even further behind us in the years to come.

QUESTION: Do you have professionals at your rap sessions?

WILLIAMS: Our rap sessions are informal. We do not have a professional present. That is the way the group wanted it. This gives parents opportunities to air their feelings, whatever they may be, without feeling threatened or intimidated. This gives us an opportunity to work with the parents to help them. You sit in the physician's office and he tells you all this stuff and at the end he says, "Do you have any questions?" If you do not have a certain amount of knowledge, you cannot ask anything. We give parents some background; we say what kinds of things are good to ask and what kinds of things parents need to know about their child's care.

COMMENT: We have a neonatal support group for parents in our unit. Because we have a limited number of physicians who are involved, we do not ask the physicians to come to the meetings. We believe also that parents who have a situation like this are very angry. To have a baby who is born abnormal, for whatever reason, is a very angry situation. Most parents who have a sick child are afraid that if they express their hostility in the presence of the physician, repercussions will occur. Each meeting is attended by the parents of neonates who are currently in the unit and by at least one set of experienced parents, who usually bring their child.

We have also found that it is helpful to keep a scrapbook of pictures of babies who have been through the unit. Over the years parents send new photos and they are all placed in the scrapbook. It helps a lot to show that book when a new parent comes in with a child who has a particular situation. You show a picture, for example, of a child who had tetralogy of Fallot and was repaired and is now five years old, doing beautifully and looking normal.

QUESTION: Did you develop any strategies to cultivate the involvement of the fathers?

WILLIAMS: I have heard of and been in contact with parent groups across the United States and I hear this all the time. When we were organizing we never questioned whether fathers would come or not. We arranged evening programs because we just automatically assumed that they wanted to come, and they do.

WITTNER: I can tell you from a physician's standpoint, dealing with the chronic problem, that there are few things more frustrating than to see the mother and the child and explain things to the mother and then either to have the father call you three hours later irate about something or to have the mother go home with all of this information and, although everything was agreed, the father just destroys everything that you have told the mother. So these evening sessions have made a big difference to me in dealing with that part of the problem.

COMMENT: One of the things we do to get fathers involved is to plan conferences around the times fathers can come where decisions are going to be made. We encourage fathers from the beginning to be there when information is given. I work with the cancer unit and when a test is going to be done to determine whether cancer is present or not, a plan is made then as to when the doctor will get together with the mother and father to give the diagnosis. That gets the father involved from the beginning.

We recently started a group for fathers alone. That is a very special time for them. It allows fathers to air the particular problems that they have.

COMMENT: Just in defense of fathers. I am from British Columbia. We are the referral for the whole of the province and the Yukon. Dads cannot quit their jobs for a couple of weeks when the kids are down. So Mom comes to the weekly meetings and, if she is lucky, she may join the evening meetings. It is really hard. Staff will make conference calls but it is difficult always to get families involved and not just Moms.

QUESTION: How did you deal with confidentiality in getting that surgery schedule?

WITTNER: I must say we have a precedent-setting situation in our area in that Long Beach has one of the largest Mended Hearts groups in the country. For the most part these adult groups, which represent thousands of people who have had coronary surgery, generally have an agreement with the hospital where a hospital bulletin is sent to the group so they know which people are having surgery and they will contact the families accordingly. We went that same route: "If they get it why can't we?" But that represents another problem. It is a problem that I thought a long time about in relationship to my patients and the group. There are families whose children are taken care of by pediatric cardiologists in other parts of Southern California and there is that ongoing problem of violating confidentiality by giving out the names.

At first, we tried just having brochures available in the office. A patient would come in and the parents would get their bill and a brochure. I mention it when there is a new patient and I talk to the parents. But it is much more effective for the group to call, and gradually we have gotten to the point where we do not think too much about it unless we hear from the family. If the parents do not want it, all they have to do is say "No." I really do not think I am necessarily violating any parents' rights by trying to provide them with a service. I do look upon this without any hesitation as an extension of my medical care because there is no doubt in my mind that it benefits the child, the parent, and me. Parents of new patients are made aware of the group and are told that we think that the group is helpful and that someone may call them from the group. If they say no, then I do not refer. There have been some people who have decided the group was not for them, they do not want the call, they do not want to have anything to do with it. And there have also been a few of those parents who have said no initially but sometime later they decide, all of a sudden, they would like to try the group.

COMMENT: A lot of parents are no longer interested in our group when they are finished with the hospital. What we have done, because we rarely get referrals, is to go to women's organizations and let them know what our services are. Some of these organizations are the La Leche League, the childbirth education groups, the nursery school parents' groups, the League of Women Voters, the American Association of University Women, or any group that deals with women who might have young children. They track you down. It is possible to locate parents out there without waiting for the hospital to refer them, if you get your information out to the other groups in the community that would possibly be involved.

unit **E**

FAMILY ADVOCACY

18

parents' advocacy
for parents

PEG BELSON

*Peg Belson, MBE, BA, is a founding member and executive board
member of the National Association for the Welfare of Children in
Hospital (NAWCH) in London, England. For many years ACCH and
NAWCH have been in close communication. Although ACCH is composed primarily of professionals, and NAWCH is composed primarily
of parents, both associations have worked to diminish the barriers to
communication between families and staff, have shared resources and
ideas and met similar obstacles in advocacy work. This paper describes
the history of NAWCH and the many contributions the organization
has made for the well-being of children and their families in health
care.*

Every year in Great Britain, three-quarters of a million children
are admitted to hospital. Yet only a little over a hundred years
ago children were grudgingly hospitalized, partly because of the
problem of cross-infection and partly because the mother was
thought to be the best possible nurse. Separation from the mother
was frowned on for, as George Armstrong, a physician with a Dis-

217

pensary for the Infant Poor, had said some years earlier, "If you take away a sick child from its parent or nurse, you break its heart immediately."

By the beginning of this century the pattern had completely changed. Children brought to hospital were usually separated from their families, sometimes for weeks. Even as recently as 1948 a child in hospital might see his parents once a week, once a month, or not at all. There were a small number of exceptions to this pattern, and it was from these and from the work done from 1948 onward at the Tavistock Institute of Human Relations on maternal deprivation and separation anxiety, that a gradual rethinking came about regarding the role of the parents—particularly the mother—in the care of the sick child.

When Professor James Spence began to admit mothers and children together to the Babies Hospital in Newcastle in 1927, he saw pediatrics as being concerned with something more than nursing and the treatment of children. It included encouraging the mother to develop her own skills by which she remains the chief instrument of child care. In 1953 James Robertson's film *A Two-Year-Old Goes to Hospital* clearly emphasized that the "greatest single cause of distress for the young child in hospital is not illness or pain but separation from mother (1) ."

THE PLATT REPORT

By 1956 sufficient concern about the need for a change in the nursing of sick children had been aroused to cause the Department of Health to set up a committee to make a special study of the arrangements made in hospitals for the welfare of ill children—as distinct from their medical and nursing treatment—and to make suggestions that could be passed on to hospital authorities. This committee's report, "The Welfare of Children in Hospital," published in 1959, has become known as the Platt Report(2) after its chairman, the distinguished surgeon Sir Harry Platt. It made a series of recommendations about the nonmedical aspects of the care of child patients in hospital, preceded by a general statement recognizing the role of the parents and the significance of the emotional and mental needs of the child.

Of the fifty-five items listed, the most significant for parents were those items that recommended that visiting to all children should be unrestricted, that provision should be made for the admission of mothers along with their children, especially children under five years of age, during the first few days in hospital. The report also advised that the trainng of medical and nursing students should include information that promotes a greater understanding of the emotional and social needs of children and their families.

The Ministry of Health adopted the Platt Report as the official policy and all hospitals were asked to implement its recommendations. But the health service did not enforce the policy. Consequently, neither change, nor understanding of the need for change, took place.

MOTHER CARE FOR CHILDREN IN HOSPITAL

In 1961 James Robertson's films were shown on television and, in a series of newspaper articles, he urged community pressure to bring about the changes that should be made in the care of children in hospital. Stimulated by the knowledge of a most pressing need, Jane Thomas, a young mother in Battersea, took his advice and called together a group of her friends to discuss the issue. Under his guidance, this group of mothers, calling itself "Mother Care for Children in Hospital," began to look into the pattern of care available in hospitals in their own district. They read books and articles and visited hospitals where unrestricted visiting and accommodations for mothers was the accepted pattern. Then they checked the pattern of visiting for local children who had been in hospital recently. These mothers visited local hospitals in which the staff had given little recognition to the Platt Report and there had been no requests by any parents for more extended visiting or for beds for mothers. Most local parents at that time saw no need for their presence in hospital when their children were admitted. The parents were, after all, handing their children over to experts. That these experts would be seen by their children as strangers was not well understood. One mother told us that she was looking forward to her children's projected visit to hospital for tonsillectomy, so that she could have a short holiday away from them. Needless to say there was no visiting for parents in that surgical ward.

The work of the new organization was to be twofold. The work was to persuade hospitals that the new concepts in child care were worthwhile and did work, and to persuade parents they had a major role to play in the care of their sick children.

Local hospital staff and parents were invited to public meetings to view and discuss the Robertson film. Senior staff members from hospitals that encouraged parental participation supported the group members. Talks were given to women's groups to publicize the work of the association and to encourage mothers to think about their children's need for mothering in hospital.

Discussions were held with nursing, medical, and administrative staff of local hospitals to discover why the Platt Report had not been implemented. A number of important factors emerged: It was considered natural for children to cry in hospital; tears had long been accepted as inevitable. It was believed that a child soon forgot what had happened in hospital; after all, his memory was very short, so no permanent damage could result. Many children who cried bitterly when they were first left, settled down and could even become quite happy. They just "didn't miss their mothers." These myths had a tenacious hold in the hospital. They were difficult to dispel.

There were other reasons given for clinging to the traditional arrangements. Some typical examples included:

- Little space to spare in the old buildings.
- Cross-infection might increase.
- The routine would be disturbed.
- Many children were in hospitals far from their parents so could not have regular visits. They would suffer if others had frequent visitors.

- Mothers would be "difficult."
- Few mothers had asked for longer visiting hours or beds in order to be with their children.
- Mothers all had home commitments that would prevent their accepting the opportunity to spend more time with their sick child.
- Since parents had not sought the changes, they would not use them if they were given.

Thus the need for change went unrecognized or was thought to be exaggerated or mistaken. The group members, however, took their message to the hospital staff in their local area. Fortified by their reading and experience of enlightened hospital care, they discussed children's needs rationally and constructively.

Publicity in the national press and in women's magazines soon stimulated the formation of other Mother Care groups. By 1962, ten groups had emerged and, following some very sympathetic coverage in the *Guardian* by Mary Stott, this number grew to thirty before the end of the year.

MOTHER CARE SURVEY

The first "Survey of Visiting," carried out by post in 1962 and supplemented by information from the thirty groups, gave details on which the Hospital Information Service was based, a service that has been extended throughout the years to cover the whole country.

This first survey showed a very wide range, both in the hours of visiting allowed and in the interpretation of "unrestricted." There were indeed some hospitals that did welcome parents throughout the day but most did not, and accommodations for mothers to live in the hospital were rarely available. One Regional Health Board advised that almost all hospitals in the Region had implemented visiting "as recommended in the Ministry of Health Circular," while the hospitals themselves reported visiting only in the afternoons, ranging from half-an-hour to a maximum of five hours. One interesting feature from a number of hospitals was that "fathers could visit in the evenings" usually from 6:00 to 6:30 P.M.

Mother Care contacted the Ministry of Health and Members of Parliament, some of whom were beginning to ask questions in the House of Commons on our behalf. Links were established with individual pediatricians, matrons [nursing supervisors], ward sisters [head nurses], and social workers, as well as with a number of voluntary and professional associations interested in the welfare of children.

SUPPORT OF PROFESSIONALS

By now it was clear that the organization needed to speak with one voice to the Ministry of Health, to the professional associations, and to the media, in order to discuss major issues and to help determine future policy. In 1963 the first national conference was convened to form a national association. The presentation to a multidisciplinary audience of current issues relating to the needs of sick children at this first conference set the pattern for future annual meetings. Dr. Dermod MacCarthy revealed that in his many years of admitting mothers and children to hospital that he had not met any difficult mothers, only difficult situations, and he maintained that staff must learn why some mothers found the hospital situation difficult and learn how to help them. James Robertson saw the organization as a meeting place for parents and hospital staff who have a common concern for the well-being of the child patient. Dr. David Morris emphasized the need to convince mothers of the value of their presence in hospital, and Barbara Weller described her children's ward where mothers— and on one occasion, a father—slept on chairbeds, and all members of the family except the dog were welcome visitors.

NAWCH IS BORN

In 1965 the organization originally called Mother Care for Children in Hospital became the National Association for the Welfare of Children in Hospital (NAWCH), a name more suited to its changing membership, since an increasing number of professional staff, pediatricians, doctors, nurses, hospital administrators, social workers, play workers, and hospital teachers joined the ranks. The work continued to expand, with local groups in most cases finding it possible to work in constructive and cooperative ways with hospitals to acknowledge the common concern of parents and staff regarding what is best for patients and families.

In 1964, NAWCH members met with the Parliamentary Secretary to contest the Minister of Health's optimistic statement in the House of Commons that "seventy-five percent of hospitals with children's wards had unrestricted visiting, by which is meant visiting by the parents at any reasonable hour of the day." NAWCH provided substantial evidence, garnered in their recent survey, that unrestricted visiting existed in only twenty-six percent of the wards. This discrepancy was caused by the fact that NAWCH inquiries were made at the ward level, while the Ministry got its figures from the hospital authorities. For NAWCH "unrestricted" meant from 10:00 A.M. to 6:00 P.M. with a one-and-a-half hour rest period excluded, a total of forty-five hours per week, while the Ministry attached no specific meaning to the term. Subsequently, the Association pressed for a clearer definition with the following results:

- In 1964, the Minister of Health explained that "unrestricted visiting meant that visitors are allowed into the ward at any reasonable hour during the day, subject to the discretion of the consultant in charge and the ward sister."
- In 1965 he explained that "reasonable hour" meant "during the hours at which children are not normally put to bed."
- In 1966, as a result of further pressure for a clear definition, the position was further clarified by the publication of *Visiting of Children in Hospital,* which stated that fixed visiting hours were

to be abandoned, that there should not be any rule restricting visiting before or after any operation, or of children who have had an infectious disease, that a decision to advise a parent not to visit a child on a particular day should be made only by the consultant physician in charge, that hospital leaflets and notices should make it clear that parents may visit at any time during the day, and that mothers of young children should be able to stay in hospital with their children.

• Later in 1966 this was followed by a request to all hospital authorities to confirm its implementation.

This precise official clarification of the position greatly helped NAWCH in its campaign to get its ideas more generally accepted both by the hospital staff and by parents. One of the problems had always been that, without evidence of official recognition, parents were reticent in pressing their needs. We could now give them this official support.

By 1967 NAWCH was an expanding organization with fifty-five groups in England and Scotland and, with a grant from the Sembal Trust, a small office was opened in London. The NAWCH *Hospital Admission* leaflet was published to alert parents of the need to be with their children in hospital and to give them the detailed information needed to help them to prepare their children for hospital. These leaflets were sold to hospitals to give to parents; by now orders for leaflets have reached half a million. For the children themselves, Ruislip NAWCH produced a comic *Simon Goes to Hospital* and Birmingham NAWCH produced *A Hospital Painting Book*. Posters, leaflets, and news-letters were developed that have helped to change public opinion and have provided teaching aids for students in many fields of child care. Slides were produced by Blackheath and Chelsea NAWCH, and films were made by various television producers and independent filmmakers.

In his 1970 revision of *Young Children in Hospital,* James Robertson(3) praised our Association for its efforts to change the quality of care for children in hospital, and he sought financial recognition for our work. The publication of *Children in Hospital: The Parents' View* by Ann Hales-Tooke(4) in 1973 emphasized the relevance of parents and gave our work and our name a welcome boost.

RELATIONSHIP TO GOVERNMENT

When unable to persuade hospitals to make the recommended changes in visiting arrangements, NAWCH has sought the help of the Department of Health and Social Security, since its principal aim is the implementation of government policy as spelled out by the Platt Committee.

Though it has received and appreciated continued support from the Department, the Association has remained a lively critic when the Department accepts the claims of hospitals that are not borne out by actual ward practice. Successive Ministers of Health have received NAWCH delegations, participated in NAWCH conferences, acknowledged the value of NAWCH work, praised "its careful fact-finding, the sense of responsibility which governed its approach, and its persistence in following up cases where it thought the practice was wrong." The Ministry acknowledged the vital role NAWCH has played in spreading information about the care of children in hospital and in keeping the Department informed about "the needs of the community at the grass roots."

In 1970 the Minister of Health appointed six members of NAWCH to Regional Hospital Boards, and in 1971 a NAWCH member was included in the Expert Group set up to look at play provision in children's wards. In 1974 changes in the structure of the Health Service brought into being a new consumer body to represent the patient—the Community Health Council—and NAWCH members were elected to many of these positions.

The Department has consulted NAWCH on a number of specific issues and its contribution to the Committee of Enquiry on Child Health Services has been particularly acknowledged. The NAWCH *Survey of Visiting Facilities and Play Provision* was published in 1973 as an appendix to the *Report of the Expert Group on Play Provision.*

Since 1971 the Department has provided financial support and in 1975 the association was able to appoint development officers in four areas where major changes were needed in the pattern of care for children in hospital.

NAWCH SURVEYS

Regular surveys of visiting arrangements and parents' accommodations have been made. In 1964 when forty-five hours was an acceptable minimum for weekly visiting, the survey found only twenty-six percent of the hospitals in one region permitted such unrestricted visiting. In 1966 only forty-five percent of the hospitals permitted unrestricted visiting and mothers were offered accommodations in only half-a-dozen of the fifty-six hospitals admitting children. By 1969 this proportion had increased to fifty-seven percent. Still, fewer than half the hospitals offered any accommodation for mothers and only in a small number of these was it offered routinely. No morning visiting was permitted in more than one-quarter of the hospitals. Our 1971 surveys showed the severely limited visiting policies of the past to be on the wane. Most hospitals offered at least five hours visiting a day, and more than three-quarters permitted visiting throughout normal waking hours. Accommodations for mothers, however, were still very limited.

By then we had raised our sights and encouraged hospitals to emulate the best. We pressed for visiting at any time of the day or night, a state of affairs we describe as twenty-four hour visiting. By 1975 this was allowed in more than a quarter of the hospitals, and in one health region by 1979 two-thirds of the hospitals offered parents visiting at any time they wished to come.

The increase of liberal visiting in general children's wards, however, was not available to children in the majority of surgical wards, particularly for children undergoing ear, nose and throat, or eye surgery. Here, visiting on the day of the operation was unusual and accommodations for mothers was virtually unobtainable.

Accommodations for parents to live in the hospital have now increased dramatically from those very limited arrangements in 1962 to some beds being available in half the wards in 1975 and in almost all the hospitals in one health region in 1979. Wards that routinely offer parents accommodations with their children find that about one-third accept, with the greatest number living-in being twenty-seven for a thirty-two bed ward.

Similar improvements have been made recently in the visiting of surgical patients, the majority of the pediatric wards are admitting parents to visit their children both before and after an operation.

Some departments have been slower to change, for example, isolation, burns and plastic surgery units, orthopedic wards, accident/emergency and outpatient departments. In many of these no consideration has been given to the special needs of children, quite often because these are, in fact, adult wards.

It is very much our hope that before long all children will be nursed in children's units, under the care of a pediatrician, as recommended in the Department's policy document about hospital facilities for children, which we believe we influenced.

PUBLIC AND PROFESSIONAL EDUCATION

NAWCH conferences and study days continue to draw a wide audience from the whole field of health care for children. These meetings have inspired important research projects such as a study determining the best pattern of care for young children in long-term care; an inquiry into valid indications for tonsillectomy; an investigation into the cost to parents of visiting children in hospital, published as *The Fares Inquiry;* a study of the problems of health care for children under one year of age who live in the inner city; and the development of an information leaflet from a particular hospital.

EXPANSION OF SERVICES

Over seventy locations in the British Isles now have NAWCH representation, with area organizers coordinating and focusing their endeavors. Assistance has been given over the years to a number of European and Commonwealth countries where similar associations are being organized. During the past two years groups from Holland and West Germany have visited us to gain personal knowledge of our ways of caring for children in hospital.

As well as stimulating change within their local hospitals, NAWCH groups and individual members have provided a variety of local welfare services. Many have been responsible for introducing play programs into the wards. Some groups pay the whole cost of the play provision; some staff and organize a hospital-financed program; others run voluntary programs on a regular basis. One group has helped to build a specially designed play-hut for the children of visiting mothers in the grounds of their hospital. Groups have provided after-school and holiday activity programs on the wards, play for handicapped children living at home, outpatient play sessions for children awaiting medical attention; and most groups have contributed toys and play equipment.

NAWCH groups also organize public meetings and film shows and provide speakers for other interested organizations. Transportation has been provided to enable mothers to visit their children in hospital and to take long-stay children home for the weekend. Members visit unvisited children in long-stay wards and children whose parents live far away. Many groups have raised funds to provide mothers' units and day-rooms and provide accommodations to supplement what is available in the hospital. Voluntary home-helps look after the children left at home. Guides have been provided in the outpatient departments to help parents fill in forms and find their way. Over the years, gifts to local hospitals have included hospital comics and hospital painting books; information leaflets in English and foreign languages; decorations, furnishings, and fittings for wards, mothers' units, waiting rooms, playrooms, and for casualty and outpatient departments; toys, play materials, clothes, and special equipment such as push-chairs, baby walkers, and locker bags; and gifts of money to help cover the cost of fares for parents who are visiting.

QUIET REVOLUTION FOR CHILDREN

Throughout the country NAWCH press secretaries have worked hard to gain for the association the responsible press, radio, and television coverage that has helped so much to get its ideas across to the public in general and helped to bring about a major change in thinking about a child's stay in hospital. Over the past eighteen years NAWCH has seen the realization in many wards of one of its major aims—the opportunity for parents to be with their children in hospital if they wish to do so. The years since the publication of the Platt Report have seen a quiet revolution in the attitudes and practices in many hospitals. Those hospitals with restricted visiting are now the exception rather than the rule and wards that routinely admit mother and child are more frequently found. Parents are far more aware of their child's need for continuing contact and a large number try to be with their children.

From an office in Central London, still with a relatively small staff, NAWCH operates an information and counseling service and distributes a range of publications to parents, students, and tutors. Local development officers stimulate the formation of new NAWCH groups, exert persuasive pressure on health authorities to gain full participation for parents in the health care of their children, and take part in training programs for hospital and community staff.

Although much has been achieved, there are still many areas that concern us. Children are still being admitted to adult wards with little parent involvement; they go unsupported to accident and emergency care; limited educational and play provision is made; some hospitals still lack any living-in accommodations for parents; surgery is still far too common an excuse for parent restriction; adolescent wards are rarely to be found; and far too many children are cared for by staff who are not specially trained in their care. Unaccompanied children seldom have the continuing care of one concerned person, now recognized as essential to their emotional well-being. The discontinuity of care is still a common practice in many of our children's wards. Parents can now support their children in many hospital wards but few hospitals can offer the support and counseling the parents themselves need in this unusual and disturbing situation.

PARENTS AND THE LAW

The issue of rights and authority is not one that has ever been clearly resolved. Over the years we have always advised parents that as far as we knew no one had ever been forcibly removed from the bedside of a sick child. However in 1974, Mr. Justice Cantley, in giving judgment on a case involving a child in hospital, found that while the plaintiff was in hospital she remained "in the custody" of her parents and that the hospital and the doctors caring for children in hospital were doing so "by the authority and on behalf of the parents who remained in a position to exercise powers of control should they wish to do so." From this judgment it would now appear that we have the law on our side, but over the years we have always suggested to parents that it is preferable to play down the issue. A struggle for supremacy over the recumbent body of a child is not what we want at all.

What we have done is to help to achieve a setting and an atmosphere wherein parents and staff can share in the care of sick children, each doing for the children what they are best fitted to do. We concentrate on the child's need for emotional security, a need that can only be met, especially in the case of a very young child, by the continued presence of the person with whom he has his closest emotional links. That, of course, is what NAWCH is all about.

REFERENCES

1. Robertson, J. *A two-year-old goes to hospital.* 16mm, 45 minutes. English, French, or German. London: Tavistock Clinic, 1953. New York: University Film Library.
2. Ministry of Health (Central Health Services Council). *The welfare of children in hospital: The report of the committee* (The Platt Report). London: HMSO, 1959.
3. Robertson, J. *Young children in hospital.* London: Tavistock Publications, 1970. Second Edition.
4. Hales-Tooke, A. *Children in hospital: The parents' view.* London: Priory Press, 1973.

19

influencing public attitudes

IVONNY LINDQUIST

Ivonny Lindquist, Head of Section at the National Board of Health and Welfare, Stockholm, Sweden, describes the progress made toward an understanding of the family and the implementation of family support policies in children's health care. Dr. Lindquist's writing has been translated into several languages. She is also active in organizing a Nordic Affiliate of ACCH.

I am happy to say that the situation for families in our hospitals has greatly improved, although there are colleagues in Scandinavia who are still struggling for a better understanding of the total needs of families in the hospital.

In our new Child Care Act, a pertinent section reads:

Parents should be entitled to visit their children at any time. Parents should be encouraged to stay with their children as long as possible to take part in their nursing, treatment, and play. Arrangements should be made to enable parents to spend the night at hospital together with their child, preferably sharing the room.

This Act created a new situation for many hospitals. Therefore, funds were granted to launch a campaign throughout Sweden

233

to inform the public about the needs of hospitalized children and parents and about what they are entitled to receive as a result of the new ruling. The campaign addresses responsible politicians as well as hospital administrators and hospital staff, not just including those in pediatrics but also those in the x-ray departments and other hospital areas that see children and families. Usually one-day conferences are arranged with emphasis on the importance of a friendly and welcoming environment.

A poster created to alert families to the new rulings says, "A child at hospital needs . . . parents for feeling safe."

The training manual that has been prepared for the hospital staff gives advice on helping children and parents to understand the psychological and emotional responses to hospitalization as well as the medical aspects. Parents receive illustrated information on all types of examinations and tests that the child is to undergo, such as x-ray, blood tests, catheterization, and others. The leaflets come in pads so that they are easy for the staff to distribute as needed.

The public information campaign includes a traveling exhibit that tours Sweden giving assistance and advice to hospitals and providing information and encouragement to parents to keep sick preschoolers at home and to care for them at home whenever possible rather than hospitalizing them.

Many Swedish hospitals now provide facilities for parents to stay with their children. Swedish law permits parents to take up to sixty days paid leave annually, if needed, for nursing their sick child either at home or in the hospital. If parents must hospitalize their child, part of their travel expenses for visiting their child is paid.

Our information campaign has had many encouraging results. One such result is that nowadays parents are much more readily accepted and welcomed at the hospitals to be with their children and to take part in their nursing.

20

parent power

CAROL HARDGROVE

Carol Hardgrove, MA, Clinical Professor, Department of Family Health Care Nursing at the University of California School of Nursing in San Francisco, urges staff and parents to be vigilant in protecting the gains that have been made in parent access, parent care, and participation.

Hospitals today are more responsive to parents than they were ten years ago. Still, there is a danger in taking too authoritarian a stance, whether it be toward today's mode of greater family involvement or yesterday's mode of family exclusion. Replacing the rule of "No parents are allowed to stay" with the rule "Every parent must stay" defeats some of the value of family inclusion. Both imperatives show a lack of understanding of the child's and family's needs and strengths. I remember the story of a Chicago mother who, after previous unhappy experiences of leaving her first child alone in the hospital in earlier, more restrictive days, girded her loins for a fight to stay with her fifth child who was to go into the hospital. She knew just what she was going to say and do when "they" directed her to leave. Instead she was told during the intake interview, "You do realize that you must stay with

235

your child during the entire time he is here, don't you?" and she found herself thinking "Hey, just a minute . . . shouldn't I be the judge of how long he needs me and whether or not I should stay?"

What is needed now is cooperative advocacy between parents and professionals for the benefit of both as well as for the child who is the patient.

Uri Bronfenbrenner speaks of the reasons why professionals and parents need to work together.

> What are the developmental antecedents of behavior disorders? The results of literally hundreds of investigations over the past three decades point to family disorganization. These forces of disorganization arise primarily not from within the family but from the circumstances in which the family finds itself and from the way of life that is imposed on it by those circumstances. Specifically, when those circumstances and the way of life they generate undermine relationships of trust and emotional security between family members, when they make it difficult for parents to care for, educate, and enjoy their children; when there is no support or recognition from the outside world for one's role as a parent, the development of the child is adversely affected (1).

We know that the hospital system without human caring is mindless and, like a juggernaut, can run over little children. It takes the intervention of parents and professionals working together to protect the child from the very efficiency that is essential to the functioning of the hospital. We must have efficiency, but we must have human caring. The most humane and caring of individual professionals working within the system cannot always halt the juggernaut alone. For one thing, working within the system can blind a person to the system and, for another, professionals are not always privy to the aftereffects of a child's hospitalization. There are numerous examples of this system-induced desensitization. Signs prohibit sibling visiting or state restricted visiting hours, but staff members no longer enforce the rules and so they no longer notice them but the signs remain posted on the walls. A nurse assures parents who hesitate about leaving crying children that children stop crying before parents are out the front door, yet parents can hear lonely children crying for Mommy up and down the corridors. Parents can only assume that staff are blind to the signs and deaf to the cries.

Professionals need the input of parents to enable them to see the family and the hospital situation afresh. Nurses have told me that one reward for them that helps prevent burn-out is when parents bring a former patient back to the unit to show how the child is growing and thriving, especially a child they feared would not live. Such episodes are rewarding to professionals, showing them that their services have not been in vain, and that infants and children do get well and that families can be appreciative. Without this parent involvement, nurses, physicians, social workers, and play activities staff who work long, hard hours efficiently and humanely may be isolated from the results of their good efforts.

Maintaining contact between parents and professionals can help professionals learn of posthospital effects, both positive and negative. Professionals can seek contact with parent groups so that they can learn more themelves and so that they can be more available to parents in less stressful arenas than the hospital.

Parents who speak out for children can be effective advocates for them, but many parents feel too intimidated to do so, assuming that they are neither needed nor welcomed by the hospital. Many are unaware of the research about the effects of hospitalization on their children. Professionals who are in touch with that research have a responsibility to share this information. Many parents do not know how to be both cooperative and assertive for the benefit of their children. They may hold back their support of the child and need to experience warm permission, acceptance, and offers of assistance in order to behave more naturally. A journal editorial suggests

> Allowing parents to visit, live-in or participate it not enough. They must be encouraged, supported and educated to be of the greatest possible help to the hospitalized child while also having their own needs met. . . . They must be well enough informed so that their nurturing activities will be in harmony with the requirements of the necessary medical treatment. . . . For the past century the more rapid the advance has

been in technology, the less emphasis there has been on the caring, the human aspects of medical practice. . . . It has been largely the pressure from parents that has resulted in improved practices for child care in hospitals, not action from the medical profession or associated health professionals. Further progress will result . . . only if there continues to be increased awareness and participation by consumers and patients in the design of health care practices(2).

Most of the changes have come about from parents who speak up. Their statements may reinforce a similar viewpoint held by the professional within the system. It is not that parents are the only ones who care about the child, but it is often the case that their voice makes a stronger impact. Parents can help move ahead a program that the professionals have been trying to promote without success for a long time. Administrators, doctors, nurses, social workers, and play activities staff who may share with parents a similar viewpoint need the clout that parent-consumers can provide. Without having the input of real-life stories and their outcomes reported by the parents, the professionals can be labeled "bleeding hearts" or "sentimentalists" by their less aware peers. The power that comes from organizing these parent voices is clearly evident in the work of major parent mutual-support groups such as the National Association for the Welfare of Children in Hospital (NAWCH) in Great Britain, or the Association for the Welfare of Children in Hospital (AWCH)(3) in Australia, and, in the United States, such groups as Candlelighters, Children in Hospitals, and Parents Concerned for Hospitalized Children and Parents With Hearts.

These groups and others offer networks of support for families and provide hospitals with materials that are useful in helping them modify policy. These groups work on the biggest job that faces us, that of educating the public to know what supports their children need in the hospital. It would be an impossible task for hospitals to prepare every prospective patient without parental help. In our hospital, for example, there are more than a thousand referring pediatricians. Getting materials to each of them, making sure each pediatrician passes the material on to each parent, and that each parent follows the written advice contained in the material is not a realistic goal.

Instead we must work together as individuals and in our organizations to raise consciousness about the important psychosocial issues involved in children's hospitalization.

Informed parent power is necessary not only for the establishment of new family-oriented programs but also for their continuance as well. Many wonderful programs in this country have vanished along with their funding at the end of their allotted five years. This is another reason why dedicated professionals must help the parents organize and work.

ENCOURAGING COOPERATIVE ACTION

How can professionals individually and in groups work with parents to help hospitals become or remain humane places that do not disrupt the family? One way is to place parents within the institutional power structure.

Three parents were successful in persuading a large New York hospital to form a parent advisory committee, which then approved a policy stating that parents may be with their child when tests, examinations, and procedures are performed except when there are medical or psychological contraindications. An explanation is given when parents are not permitted. The director of the division of mental health said, "I am absolutely in favor of parental presence whenever possible. The parent's role doesn't end at the hospital door." The newspaper article in which this story appeared(4) pointed out that the lack of clear policy had resulted in situations in which harried interns, residents, and nurses made decisions that they claimed were policy. But we all know that policy in any particular hospital differs according to who is speaking. When the new policy of including parents was set, the chief resident said, "This wouldn't have happened without the mothers. . . . It is an example of how communications should take place between consumers and their doctors, and it hasn't occurred often in the past. Now doctors are being educated by parents."

On the staff of that hospital there are many notable experts on early childhood, experts who are all for parents, but it took the parents to institute the policy. This underscores the fact that parents have a great deal of power if they realize it. One of the greatest helps that professionals can give parents is to help them realize their own power.

Parents also need to know and to help their children know that the professional is not an adversary or an enemy. The institution's system, being nonhuman, cannot be trusted, but parents can be trusted if they serve as advocates and protect children from being ground down by the system.

Professionals can help parents advocate appropriately for their children. Otherwise some parent behavior may seem bizarre, not only to staff but also to the parents' own children. Parents who are invited and supported, even courted, usually have a less defensive, more natural and positive style of being at home in the hospital. They feel free to continue their parenting. Having permission to be there may help them form ties with the other parents and they can then support each other.

It is too much to expect that total responsibility for psychological care should rest solely with either parents or professionals. Busy staff have their hands full with the care of very sick children. The staff cannot take on total responsibility for parent education. This is one of the great contributions of the Association for the Care of Children's ·Health. Through meetings with parent groups, nursery school, kindergarten, and parent-teacher-student associations, through programs on radio and television, we can educate our communities about children's needs and effective parent behaviors in health care. Parent groups and professional groups enhance each other's strength by conduits between them that prevent their becoming adversaries.

Parent groups are invariably eager for programs about such topics as preparation and parent involvement. Health care professionals are interested in parents' perceptions of the hospital and in the sequelae of hospital experiences. They need this feedback because children often exhibit very different behavior after they go home from that which they displayed in the hospital.

In addition to informing the public about the needs of children in hospitals, parent organizations have given hospitals a boost toward change. For example, Children In Hospitals did a survey of policy regarding parental access to their hospitalized children. Seven of the hospitals surveyed changed their position on open visiting and free access to children as a result of reading what other hospitals were doing in that realm(5).

Parents Concerned for Hospital Children wrote a position paper at the request of a Chicago hospital that was considering abolishing the pediatric unit and scattering the pediatric patients throughout the adult wards(6). After the paper was presented the hospital maintained the pediatric unit.

ACCH consultants have developed informative materials for parents, have organized conferences to inform other professionals about important psychological issues relevant to families, and have been influential in generating new parent programs.

We have a long way to go, both in mobilizing parent power and in making our pediatric units what we wish them to be and know they should be. In a recent survey of hospitals with stated policies of commitment to family inclusion, great gaps between philosophy and practice were revealed. Very few hospitals, for example, encourage or even permit parents to be with their child during the induction of anesthesia or in the recovery room. Very few employ a person with responsibility for contacting and looking after parents(7).

Even when we succeed in making changes for the better, we cannot be complacent in any area because programs can slip away unless we persevere and hang onto them. We must work with the school system as well as the health sytem, so that schoolchildren have positive experiences with health centers while they are well. Most importantly, we can work directly by sharing ideas with our colleagues, with friends and neighbors, and with our own families.

We need to root out archaic ideas and prohibitions that have done so much damage in splitting families in the past. We must be sure that we do not blindly continue policies that harm families. We have to be sensitive to the needs of families and use our knowledge of child development so that we increase and enhance the family's sense of integrity.

REFERENCES

1. Bronfenbrenner, U. Who cares for America's children? In V. Vaughan and T. B. Brazelton (Eds.), *The family: Can it be saved?* Chicago: Year Book Medical Publishers, 1976.
2. Korsch, B. Issues in humanizing care for children. *American Journal of Public Health,* 1978, *68*, 831–832.
3. McEwin, R. Policies of the Association for the Welfare of Children in Hospital from the Health Commission of New South Wales' point of view. *Journal of the Association for the Care of Children in Hospitals,* 1977, *6*, 29–30.
4. Brozan, N. Parents fought to be with children in hospital—and won. *New York Times,* September 27, 1976, page 38C.
5. Children in Hospital. *Boston area hospital survey update.* Children in Hospital, 31 Wilshire Park, Needham, MA 02192.
6. Parents Concerned for Hospitalized Children. *Your child and the hospital.* Parents Concerned for Hospitalized Children, P.O. Box 101, Lombard, IL 60148.
7. Hardgrove, C., & Kermoian, R. Parent inclusive pediatric units: A survey of policies and practices. *American Journal of Public Health,* 1978, *68*, 847–850.

21

humanizing
health care
for children
and their families

ASSOCIATION FOR THE CARE OF CHILDREN'S HEALTH

The Association for the Care of Children's Health is a multidisciplinary, international organization that promotes the psychosocial well-being of children and families in health care settings. Founded in 1965, the association now has members in the United States, Canada, and ten other countries. This paper is adapted from an ACCH statement on the family in health care.

Four-and-a-half million children are hospitalized in the United States each year; about 600,000 of them are under one year of age. Only ten percent of the children hospitalized in the United States receive care in a pediatric facility with staff who have re-

243

ceived special training in child development. The other ninety percent are treated in general hospitals, where less recognition may be given to the widely disparate emotional needs of a seven-day-old newborn, a seven-year-old child, and a seventeen-year-old adolescent.

Threats posed to the emotional security and development of many children and their families by serious illness, disability, disfigurement, treatment, interrupted human relationships, and nonsupportive environments have been demonstrated clearly by worldwide research studies. The outcomes can range from temporary, but frequently overwhelming, anxiety and emotional suffering to long-standing or permanent developmental handicaps.

A child's illness is often traumatic for parents, though illness can strengthen family relationships. Frequently, however, it places a significant burden on or even destroys the family structure. The divorce rate among parents of children with birth defects requiring long-term care is at least fifty percent. Many parents experience anxiety, guilt, or helplessness at one stage or another of their child's illness. These feelings, often combined with negative attitudes or misconceptions toward health care coming from their own childhood experiences, create an atmosphere of apprehension and distrust. As a result, parents may try to avoid health care settings as much as possible. This creates a pattern of acute, episodic visits to the emergency room, rather than the more desirable use of routine well-child care and of preventive health measures. This avoidance leads to low compliance with doctors' orders and to a continuing cycle of poor health maintenance.

Education is an excellent means of alleviating such situations. Studies indicate that children of parents who have received well-timed, adequate information adapt better than those of uninformed parents. The children recover more quickly and have fewer postoperative complications, and parents report greater satisfaction with medical care. Appropriate psychosocial support maximizes the natural resiliency of children and can enable hospitalization to become a positive, growing, and ego-enhancing experience.

Confronted with convincing studies, it becomes vitally important to direct new efforts toward humanizing health care and to make parents more sensitive to the special needs of hospitalized children and the siblings of these children. Planners and providers of medical care must realize that any illness endangers the emotional security and physical well-being of the child as well as the integrity of the family.

ACCH RECOMMENDATIONS FOR ACTION

To improve the quality of child health care for all children and to foster family strength, the Association for the Care of Children's Health presents the following recommendations:

1. Public education programs are needed to acquaint parents with the special needs of children in health care settings and to encourage efforts at the community level to humanize health care for children and their families.
2. Major attention should be given to the perinatal hospitalization experience. Educational and supportive programs are necessary to foster healthier and more normal attitudes toward pregnancy, birth, early infant management, and family needs.
3. All hospitals which admit children for any type of care should meet the following minimum standards:
   a. Pediatric facilities in urban areas should have no less than twenty beds and an annual occupancy rate no less than seventy percent. Rural child health should be centralized to a degree which offers quality pediatric services balanced with the need for accessibility and for the involvement of parents.
   b. There should be no restrictions on parent visiting hours. Hospitals should develop policies allowing siblings to visit while maintaining guidelines for proper infection control.
   c. Accommodations for a hospitalized child's parent to room in should be provided. Sleeping facilities for parents of children in intensive care or a neonatal unit should be provided within or near the hospital.
   d. Parent education programs should be expanded and

offered regularly in hospitals and ambulatory settings.
    e. Health professionals must ensure that children and
       their parents are informed, understand and are sup-
       ported prior to, during, and following experiences
       which are potentially distressing.

4. Hospitals should develop care-by-parent units which utilize parents as the primary caregiver. Such programs
   strengthen child and parent relationships, facilitate the
   transition to home care, and are cost-effective.

5. Hospitals should expand ambulatory and home care programs.

6. Development of low cost housing near health care facilities should be encouraged since these facilities reduce
   hospitalization time, expand utilization of ambulatory
   services, and reduce stress for families.

7. Hospitals should develop systems to handle certain surgical and medical procedures on a short stay or in/out basis
   thus reducing the need for overnight hospitalizations.
   The programs must be designed with the appropriate
   psychological support for patient and family.

8. Tertiary health care for children must be clearly defined
   and provided only by institutions with psychosocial support services for children and families, as well as adequate
   pediatric medical and surgical capabilities.

9. Research is needed to document further the specific requirements of children and families in health care settings, particularly from a developmental perspective.

10. Research is needed to determine new ways to increase
    patient and family compliance with prescribed treatment;
    to emphasize preventive medicine; to encourage children
    and adolescents to take an active role in their own health
    care; and to develop new ways of teaching effective pat-
    terns for parenting.

SUMMARY

Humanizing medical care must become a primary concern of today's health care provider and consumer alike. Humanizing care
for children is even more important, not only because of the vul-

nerability of the child, but also because attitudes that the child forms toward the health care system are usually maintained throughout life and are often eventually passed on to his or her children and thus affect the next generation of families.

When psychosocial support systems are built into the delivery of care and when parents are recognized as a valuable resource, physical recovery is hastened and there are fewer psychological problems. Attention to the human side of medicine must become an integral part of diagnosis and treatment. This is not just good medical practice; it is also cost effective. Humanizing medical care is preventive medicine in its finest sense.